WHY
AM I *ALWAYS* SO ?
TIRED?

ALSO BY ANN LOUISE GITTLEMAN, M.S., C.N.S.

The 40/30/30 Phenomenon

Get the Salt Out

Get the Sugar Out

Your Body Knows Best

Beyond Pritikin

Super Nutrition for Men

Super Nutrition for Women

Super Nutrition for Menopause

Guess What Came to Dinner

Before the Change

Beyond Probiotics

The Living Beauty Detox Program

WHY
AM I *ALWAYS* SO
TIRED?

*Discover How Correcting Your Body's
Copper Imbalance Can:*

—Keep Your Body from Giving Out Before Your Mind Does

— Free You from Those Midday Slumps

—Give You the Energy Breakthrough You've Been Looking For

Ann Louise Gittleman, M.S., C.N.S.

with Melissa Diane Smith

HarperSanFrancisco
A Division of HarperCollins*Publishers*

This book is dedicated to Carol Faye Templeton
whose boundless energy I wish for everyone.

A hardcover edition of this book was published in 1999 by HarperCollins Publishers.

HarperCollins Web Site: http://www.harpercollins.com

HarperCollins®, 🔥 ®, and HarperSanFrancisco™ are trademarks of Harper-Collins Publishers Inc.

HarperCollins books may be purchased for educational, business, or sales promotional use. For information please write: Special Markets Department, HarperCollins Publishers Inc., 10 East 53rd Street, New York, NY 10022.

First HarperSanFrancisco edition published in 1999.

Designed by Kris Tobiassen

Library of Congress Cataloging-in-Publication Data

Gittleman, Ann Louise.
    Why am I always so tired? : discover how correcting your body's copper
  imbalance can: keep your body from giving out before your mind does, free
  you from those midday slumps, give you the energy breakthrough you've been
  looking for / by Ann Louise Gittleman, with Melissa Diane Smith.
      p. cm.
  Includes bibliographical references
  ISBN 0–06–251569–1 (cloth)
  ISBN 0–06–251594–2 (pbk.)
    1. Fatigue—Etiology.   2. Copper—Pathophysiology.   3. Zinc—
Pathophysiology.   I. Smith, Melissa Diane.   II. Title.
RB150.F37G55   1999
616'.0478—dc21   98–45996

03 04 ❖/RRD 10 9 8 7 6 5

Contents

Acknowledgments

T he writing of a book is never easy, but this is even more true when you're writing about an underground topic such as copper overload. A great many people contributed to this book in both small and large ways. First, I'd like to thank my editor, Caroline Pincus, who believed in this book's message right from the start and saw it through to completion—and also her hard-working assistant, Sally Kim.

I'm very indebted to Melissa Diane Smith, whose diligence and passion for the topic helped to make this manuscript into a book that's straightforward, honest, and timely. I couldn't have done this without her and her unwavering commitment to the project.

I also would like to express my appreciation to the following professionals, who agreed to be interviewed and graciously shared their knowledge and expertise on copper overload: Jane Ayres, M.A., L.M.H.C.; Michael Biamonte, N.D.; Leonid Gordin, M.D.; Linda Lizotte, R.D., C.D.N.; Virginia Lucia; Rick Malter, Ph.D.; Julius Nestor; David Vaughan, N.C.; Larry Wilson, M.D.; and David Watts, D.C., Ph.D.

My clients are experts on copper overload in their own right. With their honesty and forthrightness, they provided me with an immense amount of firsthand information for which I'm truly thankful.

I'd also like to acknowledge the many supporters who helped and encouraged this book in oh-so-many ways—most especially my literary agent Michael Cohn, editor Liz Perle, managing editor Terri Leonard, copyeditor Kathy Reigstad, publicists Amy Durgan, Meg Lenihan, Karen Bouris, and Margery Buchanan, and friends and colleagues Jack Challem, Beth Salmon, Laurel Kallenbach, Holly Sollars,

Don Smith, and Stuart Sandler. Special thanks go to Stuart Gittleman, for the countless hours he spent researching the latest copper studies, and to Helen Smith, for her careful proofreading and editorial suggestions.

Finally, I feel most gratefully and sincerely indebted to Paul C. Eck and Carl Pfeiffer, M.D., Ph.D., nutritional researchers and pioneers who were the first to bring the epidemic of copper overload to light. I hope that this book does both Eck's and Pfeiffer's revolutionary work justice and brings their important message to the masses.

I will always be especially grateful to the Eck Institute of Applied Nutrition and Bio Energetics in Phoenix, Arizona for serving as a major source of inspiration to me. This institute is a warehouse of information on many aspects of copper toxicity based upon the research compiled by Paul C. Eck, a tissue expert and researcher who spent twenty-five years studying mineral levels and how they affect health.

Foreword

For the past twenty-five years I have dedicated myself to the practice of nutritional medicine. As is true in most general medical practices, a preponderance of my patients have been women—tired women.

Having immersed myself in this quarter-century quest for solutions to the chronic fatigue epidemic, I was delighted and gratified to read Ann Louise Gittleman's new book *Why Am I Always So Tired?*

Unexplained chronic fatigue is probably the main reason for the sudden popularity of alternative medicine. People are tired of being told that their fatigue is probably in their heads due to stress or psychiatric causes. In traditional medicine, if the routine physical exam and blood tests are normal, the quest to delve any deeper in to "why am I always so tired?" usually ends.

A nutritionally orientated doctor may probe into often overlooked areas like diet, food allergy, blood-sugar imbalance, vitamin, mineral, and other metabolic disorders, and adrenal glandular activity. If the patient has chronic fatigue syndrome, the investigation extends to the immune system and to any hidden sources of infection.

This book is a major eye-opener and should serve as a powerful tool in the nutritional treatment of chronic fatigue. Ms. Gittleman has put forth a rather bold and daring thesis—that "copper overload" and an imbalance in body levels of two trace minerals—copper and zinc—may be a root cause of most unexplained chronic fatigue conditions and is intimately associated with low thyroid and adrenal gland problems.

To propose that these two trace minerals are the common denominator of what makes most people tired—is startling. Yet, she develops and defends this position in a step-by-step fashion—documenting how the American public has become overloaded with copper—from copper containing pesticides used on fruits and vegetables to copper that leaches into our water supply and the shocking realization that estrogen causes our bodies to retain copper—which renders women much more susceptible to the copper assault. Environmental chemicals—which have estrogen activity—may compound that assault. Add to this another startling fact: the dietary approach many health-conscious people have adopted—with its emphasis on complex carbohy-drates and plant food and its prohibition of red meat—can *accelerate* copper overload.

It took courage and conviction for Ms. Gittleman to challenge the very diet that she championed in the early 1980s—because of its repeated connection in her research and clinical practice—as producing tired bodies with overactive minds. The book is replete with stories of tired people eating a variety of plant-based diets who could not shake their fatigue until the high-copper foods like soy (perhaps the worst offender), whole grains and avocado were reduced and zinc-rich foods consisting mostly of eggs and flesh proteins were replenished. She contends that this diet, which flies in the face of the popular lacto-vegetarian approach, restores zinc and copper to a more healthful level.

But don't be discouraged because Ms. Gittleman provides an energy revitalizing program with a variety of menu plans to transition into a diet that can maintain copper and zinc balance in the future.

For the health practitioner, the section on the proper diagnosis of zinc-copper imbalance was most helpful. Ms. Gittleman intones that it is easy to miss a diagnosis of copper overload because tissue levels of copper may be high while blood levels may be low. It takes patience and careful scrutiny of the laboratory parameters she has set forth to make the diagnosis.

Therefore, she feels that many cases of copper overload have been missed by not knowing some basic ground rules of test interpretation.

I am so intrigued by this book that I intend to search for zinc-copper imbalances in my tired patient population. This may well be a seminal book—a courageous eye-opener that could fundamentally alter our approach to the treatment of chronic fatigue.

—MICHAEL ROSENBAUM, M.D.

Preface

During the latter half of the twentieth century, a new health problem has developed, causing many people to feel fatigued. The problem—the buildup of copper in body tissues—is something most doctors know nothing about, so the condition almost always goes undiagnosed and untreated.

Many people who are tired in this day and age have no idea why they can't regain their energy. Although they may try everything from fad diets to treatments for medical conditions that are suspected as the culprits behind the tiredness, they often are baffled; nothing seems to reverse their fatigue. One of the reasons for this dilemma in many cases is that they haven't treated the real cause of their fatigue, which may be copper overload. I wrote this book for all of those people, including myself, who have been fatigued because of copper overload and haven't known the real reason why.

In Chapter 1, I'll take you through the frustration I experienced at not being able to help my clients regain their energy, and I'll explain how that frustration caused me to keep looking for the answers until I found the strong correlation between copper imbalance and fatigue.

In Chapter 2, you'll learn what most doctors know about copper and copper overload, and you'll see the new information I've discovered about how copper excess and copper-zinc imbalance can cause fatigue and other health problems. Chapters 3 through 5 explain the many reasons that fatigue from copper overload is so common. These chapters cover surprising contributors to copper-induced fatigue—everything from trendy "light" diets to widespread use of the birth control pill to excessive stress. Then, in Chapter 6, I'll show you that fatigue really is the tip of the iceberg of the many common health problems copper overload can cause. When you take steps to reverse copper overload, you can not only improve your energy but also alleviate or even eradicate numerous other health complaints in the process.

The second half of the book—Chapters 7 through 11—is devoted to showing you how you can regain your energy and health by reversing copper overload. In Chapter 7, you'll learn how you can determine if copper overload is the source of your fatigue and other health problems. Then, in Chapters 8 through 11, I'll take you step by step through the time-tested program I've developed to help individuals reverse copper overload and regain energy. The program involves diet, use of the right supplements, and stress management. It's a program I've fine-tuned over the past decade and used with great results with thousands of my clients who've had copper overload and the fatigue that accompanies it.

I've been working with individuals who've had copper-induced fatigue for more than ten years, and I know how frustrating it can be for individuals who have this condition and don't know it. If you've been discouraged by fatigue that hasn't lessened no matter what you do, take heart. If copper overload is an unsuspected factor behind the fatigue you're experiencing, I'm confident that the program I outline in this book will help you.

This book is intended solely for education and information, not as medical advice. Please consult a medical or health professional if you have questions about your health.

Part I

Searching for Answers to Fatigue

Chapter One

Uncovering the Copper Connection to Fatigue

More than a decade ago, I was beside myself with frustration in my nutrition counseling career. I couldn't get to the bottom of a mystery—the mystery of why a significant number of my clients were always so tired. I was determined to help my clients feel better, so I offered them all types of cutting-edge nutrition advice that I believed would help their energy. No matter what I tried, though, many of my clients continued to experience fatigue. This perplexed me. Becoming increasingly frustrated, I searched high and low for answers.

Fatigue is a national epidemic. Eighty percent of Americans report feeling tired most of the time. Fatigue also is a major public health problem, when you consider how it impacts our lives. When we're tired, we find ourselves less productive at work and less able to accomplish what we want to accomplish. We bow out of things we love to do with the ones we love simply because we're too exhausted. We also become irritable and depressed and unpleasant to be around. As energy doctor Michael Rosenbaum, M.D., is fond of saying, "No one is dying of fatigue, but everyone is suffering from it."

I really wanted to help my clients so that they could enjoy more fulfilled and productive lives, so I approached the fatigue problem as any health practitioner would: I looked first to all the accepted causes. Fatigue can develop because of a wide variety of factors—both medical and nutritional in nature. These include medical conditions such as hypothyroidism (low thyroid function), anemia, and depression, as well as lifestyle factors such as inadequate sleep and lack of proper nutrition. I found that some of the clients who consulted me did indeed have one or more of these underlying medical conditions, but even when such problems were medically or nutritionally treated, most of my clients *still* didn't find themselves regaining their vim and vigor. Disappointed and baffled, I kept asking myself why.

In numerous other cases, there was no apparent reason that my clients should be fatigued. In assessing these clients, I ruled out common medical causes and looked further to diet and lifestyle. (I usually can quickly identify unhealthy eating and lifestyle habits that undermine energy levels, because I've been a nutritionist for more than 20 years.) But I didn't see any of the obvious mistakes that many people make. The men and women who came to see me were intelligent and health-conscious; they were doing virtually everything right—eating nutritious, light meals frequently, taking broad-spectrum nutrient supplements, and trying to get enough sleep and rest. Some were meditating or practicing stress reduction on a daily basis. Yet in spite of all their efforts, they inexplicably felt sapped of energy. I wasn't quite sure what to tell them. I offered them a wide variety of up-to-date nutrition advice that I thought would help their energy level, but none of my suggestions worked. This confounded me, testing my ability as a nutritionist, so I kept searching for solutions.

After much investigation and analysis, I eventually discovered that the answer to my clients' fatigue didn't involve any of the well-accepted causes: it was a case of simple nutritional imbalance. If I'd known where to look during those early years of frustrated searching, the nutritional imbalance that was behind so much of my clients' fatigue would have been relatively easy to detect and correct. (You'll learn how you can do that for yourself later in this book.) But I didn't look in the right places, at least not initially. Like many practitioners, I based my advice on my nutrition education, my medical knowledge and interpretation of standard medical tests, and my ability to stay on top of the results of the latest scientific research. These skills didn't help me uncover the answer, however. To crack the code of the missing link to fatigue, I had to follow my gut instincts, use an unconventional diagnostic tool, and analyze the clinical picture that presented itself among the clients in my practice. The following case studies will show you how that picture unfolded in three clients—a picture that spurred me on to find a common, unsuspected, and easily treatable cause of fatigue.

WHEN TREATING HYPOTHYROIDISM DIDN'T BOOST ENERGY

Jennifer

Jennifer, a 31-year-old advertising copywriter, told me when she came into my office that she was exhausted—and she looked it. "I think there's some reason why I'm so tired, but I've seen five different doctors and been tested for everything from anemia to the Epstein-Barr virus. All of the tests have showed up negative," she said, her voice cracking. "Some of the doctors I've seen have insinuated that I might be a hypochondriac. I don't think I am, but I'm starting to wonder."

I could see the desperation in her face and hear it in her voice as she talked slowly and methodically. I asked her to tell me more about her fatigue and the other symptoms she was experiencing. "Well, I have a hard time getting out of bed in the morning," she said, "and I need several cups of coffee to feel even somewhat alive. It seems as if my body is always cold and my skin is dry, no matter how much moisturizer I put on it. I've also been steadily gaining weight over the last several years, and I'm frequently constipated. I'm also often depressed, but I think my depression stems from feeling so tired and lousy."

After hearing Jennifer's story, I deduced that one of her problems might be low thyroid function, which is a common cause of fatigue. She told me she'd had standard thyroid profile tests run many times, and they'd all come out normal. But I asked her to perform a more sophisticated diagnostic screening tool—the Barnes basal temperature test—on her own. (This test involves shaking down a thermometer as far as it will go before you go to sleep at night and putting it beside your bed. When you wake up in the morning, before getting out of bed, you place the thermometer under your armpit and lie quietly for ten minutes before reading the thermometer.) Jennifer performed this test repeatedly and told me the results the next time I saw her: an underarm temperature consistently below 97.8 degrees. This is usually a sign that subclinical hypothyroidism is present—which was exactly what I was expecting.

I set to work advising Jennifer on steps she could take to boost her thyroid function, emphasizing increasing her intake of thyroid-essential iodine by taking kelp tablets and eating more seafood. She told me that following this advice would be easy for her because she loved shellfish.

I continued to see Jennifer every few weeks. She followed my advice to a T and loaded up on shellfish and kelp supplements. But as the months went by, she reported to me that her fatigue, constipation, and depression not only continued but actually became worse. She also developed new symptoms, including anxiety and insomnia. This baffled me.

Numerous questions ran through my head. *If low thyroid function is behind Jennifer's fatigue and she's taking steps to boost thyroid function, why isn't she feeling more energetic? Why are these new symptoms developing? What exactly is going on here?* I reasoned that there must be another factor involved in this case, something I was missing, so I went looking for more clues.

Blood tests sometimes disclose gross mineral deficiencies that cause fatigue, so I encouraged Jennifer to have a blood nutrient profile performed. She agreed to have that test done, and I was eager to see the results. To my dismay, however, they revealed nothing unusual. Frustrated, I wondered how I should proceed.

I'd tried most of the standard and well-accepted diagnostic tools available, so I decided to try something unconventional and not as widely accepted: tissue mineral analysis. I knew from my nutrition training that heavy metals such as lead and mercury sometimes build up in tissues and cause fatigue and other far-reaching health problems. I also was aware that tissue mineral analysis was accepted by the Environmental Protection Agency as a way to test for toxic metal exposure. It seemed reasonable to me that this test might give some clues to Jennifer's health puzzle.

I expected to see a high level of some obscure toxic metal on the tissue mineral analysis, but that didn't happen. The only abnormality I saw on the test results was a high level of copper. Copper performs many critical functions in the body, so I saw the high copper level as an interesting but insignificant sidelight; I didn't think much about it. I had no idea then that the high copper level on Jennifer's tissue test would be the beginning of a pattern—a pattern that would help me identify an overlooked cause of fatigue.

WHEN TREATING ANEMIA DIDN'T BOOST ENERGY

Ellen

During the same time period I was counseling Jennifer, I started working with Ellen, another client who complained about exhaustion. When Ellen came into my office, I saw that she was a pretty, 40-year-old woman who would have been a lot more attractive if her skin hadn't been so pale. "I feel physically wiped out all the time," she began, "and I experience heavy bleeding during my menstrual period. I also feel too weak to exercise and have frequent headaches." The symptoms she was experiencing, along with the pallor of her skin, suggested anemia as a cause for her fatigue, so I asked her to see her doctor to have the appropriate tests for this condition performed. The tests revealed what I was expecting: iron-deficiency anemia.

Two of the best ways to help the body overcome iron-deficiency anemia and the fatigue that accompanies it are to take blood-boosting nutrient supplements that contain iron, copper, vitamin B-12, and folic acid, and to eat iron-rich liver at least twice a week. I suggested these measures to Ellen, and she agreed to try them.

Several months went by before Ellen called me for another appointment. Confident that my nutrition suggestions had helped improve her energy, I assumed that I hadn't heard from her because she was doing well. When she stepped into my office, she didn't look very healthy, but I still expected good news when I asked her how she was doing.

"Not well," she said, taking a seat.

"Why not?" I asked, surprised and concerned.

"I'm more tired and depressed than ever, and my headaches have gotten worse, especially right before my period. I'm so tired that I become panicky and get irritable with those I love every time any extra stress comes into my life. I'm pretty discouraged that I'll ever be able to feel healthy, energetic, and well balanced again. What's wrong with me?"

Ellen's impassioned cry for help struck a chord with me, and I was determined to help her find answers. Remembering that heavy metals can be the unsuspected culprits behind exhaustion, I suggested that Ellen have a tissue mineral analysis performed. She agreed.

When the results of Ellen's test came back, I checked the levels of toxic metals such as lead and mercury. They were all low. Another dead end, I thought. But then I looked at the rest of the chart and saw a high level of copper, just as I had on Jennifer's chart. Copper again. *Could there be anything wrong with too much copper?* The seed of that intriguing question eventually grew in my mind. Initially, however— although it occurred to me that there might be some connection between copper and fatigue—I had no idea what a high level of copper meant.

WHEN NO MEDICAL CAUSE FOR FATIGUE COULD BE FOUND

Joyce

Immediately after meeting with Ellen for the first time, I saw Joyce, a 25-year-old artist who had a sweet, sensitive nature and a thin (almost gaunt) appearance. Like Jennifer and Ellen, Joyce came to see me because she suffered from fatigue and didn't have any idea why.

"I started feeling tired several years ago and saw numerous conventional doctors and specialists. They tested me for everything from anemia to parasite infections," Ellen explained. "None of them found anything wrong with me, though, so I got discouraged with conventional medicine and started trying natural remedies on my own and seeing alternative practitioners." Joyce told me she had first consulted an Oriental medical doctor who performed acupuncture on her over several sessions. Then she had turned to a homeopathic practitioner who prescribed individualized remedies and a naturopathic doctor who tailored a diet for her. She also read a book discussing how important minerals are for health and, consequently, began taking megadoses of multimineral complexes. "Some of these things made me feel worse and others seemed to help momentarily, but none of them really got at the root of my fatigue and helped me regain my energy," she said.

Nutrition is my forte, so I asked her about her diet. "About a year after I began to feel especially tired, I switched to a low-fat, whole-food, mostly plant-based diet at the suggestion of the naturopathic doctor I consulted. He convinced me that this type of diet would help increase my energy," she explained. "I believed him, but I think that was wishful thinking. After a while, I just began to feel worse—like my body and mind were out of balance. My mind was always active with a lot of creative ideas, but my body felt burned out."

After hearing Joyce's story, I suspected that her diet needed more balance and advised her to emphasize a little more healthy fat, in the form of nuts and avocados. I also asked her if she'd consider having a tissue mineral analysis performed. Although Joyce had already had countless other tests performed by doctors, a tissue mineral analysis is the only reliable test that reveals heavy metals in the tissues, and it's affordable. I explained this to her, and she agreed that the test was worth trying.

The results of the test came back in a week or so. I opened up the envelope, pulled out the chart, and glanced over the results quickly. What did I see? A high copper level. *Hmm,* I thought, *there's that copper again. Is this test trying to tell me something?*

SEEING THE CONSISTENT PATTERN

Jennifer, Ellen, and Joyce taught me many lessons, although they probably didn't know it. Unfortunately and regrettably, I made a number of mistakes in giving advice to each one because, like many practitioners, I didn't know anything about the connection between high tissue copper and fatigue. These three women were of different ages and different lifestyles and appeared to have unrelated health problems, but all three shared two common bonds: feeling tired most of the time and having a high tissue copper level. After linking the high copper levels in their cases, I began to ask myself, *Is there some missing link between copper and fatigue that most practitioners are missing?* To gain more evidence and help find answers for still other clients who were frustrated by unexplained fatigue and other baffling symptoms, I began advising more and more of my clients who didn't respond to conventional ways of overcoming fatigue to have a tissue mineral analysis performed.

Even though I was curious about what a string of tissue mineral analyses would reveal over time, I wasn't really expecting to see a consistent pattern. One by one, though—over and over again—I did. No matter how the individual cases of hard-to-treat fatigue varied in other specifics, *copper imbalance showed up eight times out of ten.* Here's a quick rundown of some of the vastly different cases I encountered:

Steve, a 51-year-old architect, complained of fatigue that he believed was caused by a mild case of hepatitis he'd had several years before. I advised him to take milk thistle, an herb known to help rejuvenate and protect liver function. This did indeed improve his liver function, allowing him to regain some energy. But he was still tired, so I suspected that a heavy metal might be a hidden culprit behind his condition. To rule out such toxicity, Steve underwent tissue mineral analysis, and high copper showed up.

Candice, a 35-year-old sculptor, regularly saw a therapist because she had a history of both emotional and physical highs and lows. Candice told me that her physical fatigue and roller-coaster emotions had become particularly pronounced shortly after she'd begun taking birth control pills seven years earlier. I convinced Candice to try tissue mineral analysis and found her tissue copper level off the chart.

Mike, a 24-year-old musician, told me that although he'd enjoyed hiking and other outdoor sports most of his life, he didn't feel like working out anymore. He explained that his fatigue and apathy had first appeared a few years after he moved to a copper-mining area of the country. Suspecting that his tissue copper level might have risen in this new environment, I encouraged him to have an analysis conducted. Once again, a high copper level was revealed.

TRYING TO MAKE SENSE OF THE PATTERN

My clinical experience was showing me loudly and clearly the strong association between fatigue and a high tissue copper level—or *copper overload,* as I began to call it. But with the little I knew about copper, my mind couldn't fit all the pieces of the puzzle together. I couldn't understand what a high copper level meant, how it was related to fatigue, or how I could help my tired clients. Over the next several months, I studied all the information about copper that I could find, reacquainting myself with basic information that I'd covered in my nutrition training and exploring avant-garde concepts about copper overload from nutrition pioneers Carl C. Pfeiffer, Paul C. Eck, Larry Wilson, and David Watts. The next chapter will give you a rundown of both the traditional and the enlightened views of copper's role in human health and energy.

Chapter Two

Basics of Copper and Copper Overload

Copper is a mineral essential for health. As a nutritionist, I of course knew this as I read my various clients' tissue mineral analyses, so I initially didn't think high copper levels were problematic. But I learned through my investigation that copper is a double-edged mineral: it performs many critical functions in the body, but it also can build up in tissues and drain energy just as heavy metals such as mercury or lead do—metals that we all know to be dangerous.

To understand the copper connection to fatigue, let's begin with some basics about copper:

> As a constituent of numerous important enzymes in the body, copper is involved in everything from energy production to pigment formation in hair and skin. It's essential for building collagen, the matrix necessary for strong bones, joints, and connective tissue; for forming hemoglobin and red blood cells; and for synthesizing neurotransmitters that send messages throughout the nervous system and brain. Copper also plays important roles in reproduction and pregnancy and in the proper function of the thyroid and adrenals, which are key energy-producing glands in the body.

We ingest copper in the foods we eat. Our bodies then absorb and utilize this copper to perform all the various functions listed above. Food sources particularly rich in copper include nuts, whole grains, soy products, organ meats, and shellfish.

The liver plays a vital role in maintaining copper homeostasis in the body, although many of the precise details of liver function still are not known. Generally speaking, when copper is ingested or is absorbed through the lungs or skin, the liver takes copper up and attaches it to copper-binding proteins that allow the mineral to be safely transported through the bloodstream so that it can perform its various functions.

Excess copper not needed by the body is normally eliminated primarily via bile, which flushes from the gallbladder through the liver into the stool. Any reduction in bile function, liver function, or gallbladder function limits the body's ability to excrete copper, causing a buildup first in the liver, then in other organs such as the brain, heart, kidneys, and adrenal glands.

As crucial as copper is, we need just a pinch of it in our bodies. The average person ingests 2.5 to 5.0 milligrams of copper per day; those who eat vegetarian and other high-fiber diets typically take in more. The range of dietary copper considered safe and adequate to meet our needs is 1.5 to 3.0 milligrams per day; the recommended daily allowance for adults is 2.0. While probably only 30 to 50 percent of the copper we take in from our diet is absorbed, most of us are exposed to considerable additional copper from environmental sources. These environmental sources will be covered in detail in Chapter 4.

If we take in too little copper or if our bodies don't absorb copper properly, the resulting low levels can lead to rheumatoid arthritis, high cholesterol, multiple sclerosis, and lowered immunity.

If we take in too much copper or if our bodies don't excrete excess copper properly, high levels can build up in the body and interfere with the action of many other nutrients, leading to overall tiredness. The nutrient that's most affected by high levels of copper is copper's primary antagonist or competitor, zinc.

THE IMPORTANCE OF COPPER-ZINC BALANCE

Copper and zinc tend to work in a seesaw relationship with each other in the body. When the levels of one of these minerals rise in the blood and tissues, the levels of its counterpart tend to fall. Ideally, copper and zinc should be in a 1:8 ratio in favor of zinc in the tissues. But stress, overexposure to copper, or a low intake of zinc can throw the critical copper-zinc balance off, upsetting normal body functioning. Even if a person's copper levels aren't unusually high, if there's more copper in relation to zinc in the tissues than there should be, fatigue can result.

THE MANY WAYS COPPER-ZINC IMBALANCE CAN CAUSE FATIGUE

Copper and zinc are found in virtually every cell, tissue, and organ throughout the body, and the body needs all cells, tissues, and organs to be functioning at peak capacity in order to produce maximum amounts of energy. When copper and zinc are out of balance at the cellular level, cells, tissues, and organs won't function optimally and the body's production of energy therefore diminishes. The following are some of the key ways copper-zinc imbalance can contribute to fatigue.

Hypothyroidism

The thyroid is one of the two main energizing glands in the body. (The other one is the adrenal glands.) The thyroid produces thyroxin (T4), a hormone that regulates energy metabolism (or, in other words, determines the rate at which the body burns food for energy). Before T4 can be used in the tissues, however, the body has to convert it into tri-iodothyronine (T3), which is the active intracellular thyroid hormone that stimulates energy-burning within the cell. Copper-zinc imbalance can impede the conversion of T4 to T3, resulting in hypothyroidism at the cell level even in people whose thyroid hormone levels are shown by blood testing of the most sophisticated type to be normal. This cell-level hypothyroidism results in slower energy production, which we experience as fatigue.

Adrenal Insufficiency

The adrenal glands—our so-called stress glands—secrete adrenal cortical hormones (chiefly cortisol), which help the thyroid hormone stimulate the energy metabolism of the body. During periods of stress, the adrenals release large amounts of these hormones to enable the body to produce more glucose—ready-to-use fuel—for the quick energy it requires. Zinc is needed for the production of adrenal cortical hormones, so if zinc levels are low or if copper levels are high, production of adrenal cortical hormones diminishes. The adrenals then aren't able to rise to the challenge of stressful situations and give the body the get-up-and-go it needs.

Liver Troubles

Copper-zinc imbalance also affects the liver, which is the main organ of detoxification in the body. Copper and zinc are both needed to activate enzymes necessary for normal liver function and detoxification, so if copper and zinc are out of balance, the ability of the liver to eliminate toxins, including excess copper, can become diminished. When excess copper is retained, other liver troubles can arise, including a slowdown of the liver in converting stored fuel (glycogen) to glucose for energy. This can be a major cause of fatigue.

Diminished Energy Production Within Cells

To provide the body with energy, the cells break down nutrients in a process called *oxidation* or *cellular respiration*. Copper and zinc are both involved in this process, so an imbalance in these minerals can interfere with the production of energy. Balance is the key here: a trace amount of copper is needed in the final stage of the production of energy—the electron transport process, through which most of the energy is generated in your cells—but too much copper can result in diminished energy production.

Tissue mineral experts have seen the strong correlation between fatigue and copper overload for decades, but copper overload as a cause of fatigue is missed by most practitioners. To understand why, you need to know how most doctors view copper overload.

COPPER OVERLOAD: THE TRADITIONAL VIEW

In traditional medical circles, only two types of copper toxicity are readily accepted and recognized: acute copper poisoning and Wilson's disease. Acute copper toxicity occurs when food or drink contaminated with high amounts of copper—vinegar-containing foods or acidic beverages like cider stored in copper vessels, for example—is ingested. This toxicity results primarily in vomiting and diarrhea—means by which the liver tries to eliminate the excess copper quickly. Prompt vomiting and diarrhea generally protect a person who's been poisoned with copper from more serious systemic effects, but not always. If the exposure to copper is too great, red blood cells can actually rupture en masse, and death can result. Rest assured, though, that this is extremely rare.

Unlike acute copper poisoning, Wilson's disease is a chronic form of copper overload. It's a hereditary disorder that causes copper to accumulate in tissues and produce extensive damage. In this disorder, a genetic defect prevents the liver from secreting copper into the blood or excreting it into the bile. As a result, the copper level in the blood is low, but copper builds up in the liver, causing cirrhosis, and then spills over into other organs, such as the eyes and brain. Treatment of the disease needs to be lifelong and requires consistent, periodic monitoring by a physician.

The conditions of acute copper poisoning and Wilson's disease illustrate quite dramatically that *too much copper can be hazardous to one's health*. However, these conditions represent two extremes that affect a very limited number of people. The average person with copper overload doesn't experience the symptoms and long-term effects of acute copper poisoning or Wilson's disease; he or she experiences a subtle degree of copper overload that most doctors aren't trained to recognize.

COPPER OVERLOAD: THE ENLIGHTENED VIEW

Most cases of copper overload, falling somewhere in the broad spectrum of subtle to mild to severe, don't fit neatly into the existing, narrow medical guidelines. Though I learned this only about ten years ago, a few savvy, holistic practitioners have known it for more than 20 years. As far back as the early 1970s, nutritional pioneers such as the late Carl Pfeiffer, Ph.D., M.D., warned that copper overload is more common than doctors recognize.

The primary symptom that individuals with copper overload notice is fatigue. As I explained earlier, any time copper builds up, the functioning of the liver, thyroid, and adrenal glands become suppressed, and tiredness can result from any one of these consequences. But fatigue really is only the tip of the iceberg, as you'll read in Chapter 6. With copper overload, fatigue usually is accompanied by a gamut of other hard-to-pin-down symptoms that women especially often complain about but seem to be able to get little relief from—everything from mental racing and insomnia to premenstrual syndrome.

SIMILARITIES BETWEEN COPPER AND IRON

Copper overload as a cause of fatigue and other health problems hasn't been recognized by most doctors, but I can assure you it will be. Although the consequences and prevalence of copper overload may seem a bit hard to believe at first, the situation with copper now is similar in many ways to that of iron several years back. Iron, like copper, is known to be an essential mineral. Indeed, a decade or more ago, most health professionals thought people couldn't get enough of it. Iron was added to many foods, including enriched breads, cereals, and flour, and routinely added in significant amounts to most supplements. Now, however, it's been well established that too much iron can lead to iron overload, a condition that can cause everything from fatigue and depression to liver dysfunction and heart disease. Most men and postmenopausal women today are advised to avoid iron supplements unless iron deficiency is confirmed. The main way to lose extra iron is with blood loss, so only premenopausal women, with their menstrual periods, are likely to be deficient; men and postmenopausal women, on the other hand, are more at risk for iron overload.

A similar situation now exists with copper, but there are several key differences. As with iron in its heyday, copper is routinely added to supplements these days, and sometimes to foods; and most of us are following today's prevalent nutrition advice to eat more plant foods (most of which, because they're quite high in copper, and often low in zinc, contribute to copper overload). But—and here's where the analogy with iron breaks down—we're also exposed to a significant amount of copper from environmental sources: we regularly ingest remnants of the fungicide copper sulfate on our produce, for example, and we consume copper as it leaches from antiquated copper pipes into the water we drink and cook with. Another difference that exists between copper and iron overload is that premenopausal women (and postmenopausal women who take estrogen replacement therapy) are the most at risk for copper overload. This is because the female hormone estrogen increases copper retention in the body. So while men and postmenopausal women need to be aware of their greater susceptibility to iron overload, premenopausal women should be making sure that they don't get too much copper.

The similarities between iron and copper aren't surprising, really. Both minerals have a great deal of electrical activity—in their ionic state they're very active metals, always searching for other molecules to react with—and therefore need to be handled very carefully by the body. If copper and iron aren't bound to proteins for safe transportation through the bloodstream, both become toxic to the body, allowing free-radical activity and damaging tissues. The body tries to guard against these consequences, but occasionally errors in the metabolism of these minerals do occur. Some people who are exposed to too much of one of these minerals aren't able to excrete the excess, for example, while others don't make enough of the proper binding proteins. It's my hunch that still others simply absorb copper too efficiently, just as certain people absorb iron too efficiently.

You should be aware of these facts and observations but not alarmed by them. Just as individuals who have iron overload (or are prone to it) can now overcome or prevent the condition by being savvy about the risk factors and by taking appropriate corrective measures (such as giving blood regularly), individuals who have copper overload (or are susceptible to it) can overcome the condition by becoming savvy about copper. This book will teach you everything you need to know to overcome this unsuspected cause of fatigue so that you can regain your energy. By reading this chapter, you've taken the first and most important step: you've learned the basics about copper overload. The next step is to understand the many reasons copper overload develops.

Chapter Three

Unsuspected Dietary Factors Behind Fatigue

More and more of us now understand that diet is almost always in some way involved in illness, and that's the case with copper overload as well. But because research in this area is so new and so little understood, many of us unknowingly eat in a way that contributes to or exacerbates copper overload, leading to ever-lower energy levels. Diet can be a culprit whether you're a busy professional eating low-fat convenience foods on the run, a health buff eating a natural-food diet, or a recurrent dieter so concerned with your weight that you eat little food at all. To illustrate this point, let's look at five of my clients who had copper-related fatigue and other health problems and the type of diet each of them ate.

Anna, the Low-Fat, High-Carbohydrate Advocate

Anna, a 35-year-old schoolteacher, came to see me because she was tired, anxious, and frequently constipated. Juggling a family and career, she was so busy with both that she had little time to worry about food. She grabbed quick-and-easy convenience foods wherever she could find them, but she did try to watch her fat intake. A typical day's menu for her looked something like this:

- A fat-free muffin and a banana for breakfast
- A sandwich and a couple of fat-free cookies for lunch
- Pretzels and a diet soda for afternoon snack
- Pasta and a little fish for dinner
- Nonfat frozen yogurt for a nighttime treat

Anna seemed quite proud of her low-fat, high-carbohydrate diet; she thought she was doing the right thing. She had no idea why she didn't feel well eating this way.

THE TROUBLE WITH LOW-FAT, HIGH-CARBOHYDRATE DIETS

The typical low-fat, high-carbohydrate diet that Anna adopted—the diet most Americans eat today—can contribute to copper overload in several ways.

Such a diet is high in sugar and processed carbohydrates, both of which are zinc-zappers. When fat is removed from foods such as muffins and cookies, additional sugar is usually added in its place. Zinc is a nutrient critical for the body's metabolism of sugar, yet sugar is void of zinc. Therefore, to properly process the sugar we eat, the body must draw on its own stores of zinc. The more fat-free, sugar-rich products we eat, the more likely we are to develop zinc deficiency. And without adequate zinc in the body, copper tends to build up.

Like sugar, the refined white-flour products found in most high-carbohydrate diets are poor sources of zinc. In the milling of white flour, up to 80 percent of the zinc in the wheat grain is removed. Other nutrients—such as many of the B vitamins and manganese, which are important for preventing copper toxicity—also are milled out in the refining process. While a few nutrients that are stripped away are added back to white-flour products in the "enriching" process, zinc, manganese, and certain B vitamins are not. Although many Americans think loading up on carbohydrates encourages health and bolsters energy, they don't realize that the more white-flour products such as pasta, muffins, breads, and cookies they eat, the greater their likelihood of developing deficiencies of zinc, manganese, and many B vitamins. These nutrients are antagonistic to copper, so when they're lacking in the diet, copper can build up unchecked.

A high-carbohydrate diet dominated by refined white-flour products also is low in fiber, and lack of fiber encourages copper accumulation. Fiber is indigestible material found in vegetables, legumes, whole grains, and fruits, and it serves a valuable purpose: it helps move the bowels and carry toxins through the digestive tract and out of the body. When little fiber is in the diet, the bowels don't move properly, and when the bowels don't move properly, excess copper isn't eliminated efficiently.

People who strictly avoid fat usually avoid animal protein sources that contain fat, such as red meats and even poultry. These are, however, our best sources of zinc. When these foods are removed from the diet, zinc intake is low, and when zinc intake is low, copper overload is likely, as we have seen. The low protein intake in the typical low-fat, high-carbohydrate diet also presents a problem. Protein is needed to help the liver make protein carriers that allow copper to be utilized and transported properly. Without enough protein, copper can accumulate undisseminated in tissues.

Key Drawbacks of Low-Fat, High-Carbohydrate Diets

- They're low in copper-antagonistic nutrients such as zinc, manganese, and B vitamins.
- They're low in fiber, which is needed for regular elimination and copper detoxification.
- They're low in protein, which is needed to help the liver use and transport copper properly.

Like many Americans, Anna thought that avoiding animal protein and loading up on low-fat carbohydrates would promote energy and health. She didn't realize that her diet was low in fiber, protein, and many nutrients, especially zinc—all of which are needed in sufficient amounts to prevent copper overload and the fatigue that accompanies it.

Celeste, the Natural-Food Enthusiast

Celeste, a 28-year-old healthcare administrator, began her first appointment with me by saying she was just plain frustrated. She suffered from exhaustion, mood swings, difficult bowel movements, and insomnia, a symptom cluster that was a bit surprising in someone who was health-conscious and nutritionally well educated. Unlike Anna, Celeste knew the importance of fiber and a wide range of nutrients in the diet, so she strictly avoided processed foods. She ate a nutrient-dense, whole-foods diet something along these lines:

- Whole-grain cereal topped with raisins, sunflower seeds, and wheat germ for breakfast
- Fruit-and-nut trail mix in mid-morning
- A soy burger on a whole-grain bun for lunch
- Popcorn sprinkled with brewer's yeast for a snack
- Shrimp or some other shellfish, whole-wheat spaghetti, and a salad for dinner

Celeste also mentioned in passing that she drank tea and iced tea often throughout the day.

THE TROUBLE WITH MANY NATURAL-FOOD DIETS

Although healthful in many respects, many natural-food diets—Celeste's included—are top-heavy in copper. Vegetarian diets, soy-based macrobiotic diets, and shellfish-based diets are all high in copper, and Celeste's diet had components of all these. Celeste didn't know it, but she was ingesting copper morning, noon, and night, right down to the tea she drank throughout the day. To get an idea of how much copper Celeste was receiving, browse through the list below, which indicates the copper content of various common foods. (As I noted in Chapter 2, the amount of dietary copper considered safe and adequate to meet our needs is 1.5 to 3.0 milligrams per day.)

Copper Content of Various Common Foods

	(mg/100 gm)
Dried yeast	4.98
Tea	4.80
Cocoa powder	3.57
Chocolate (bitter)	2.67

Wheat germ	2.39
Sunflower seeds	1.77
Lobster	1.69
Sesame seeds	1.59
Crab, canned	1.52
Molasses	1.42
Walnuts	1.39
Ground coffee	1.26
Soybeans	1.17
Pecans	1.14
Curry powder	1.07
Chocolate (sweet)	1.04
Wheat bran	1.01
Mushrooms	1.00
Navy beans	.85
Kidney beans	.84
Peanuts	.62
Shrimp	.60

Given the amount of copper Celeste was consuming—compounded by the fact that she also was taking the birth control pill, which increases copper retention—I wasn't surprised that Celeste had typical symptoms of copper overload.

Celeste was overdosing on copper in her diet and didn't know it. She did know about the importance of zinc for health, however, and thought she was getting enough of that nutrient from the shellfish, nuts, and whole grains she ate. What she didn't realize is that while these foods contain a significant amount of zinc, they're also incredibly rich in copper; in other words, they have a poor copper-to-zinc ratio. As a result, the copper in these foods cancels out much of the zinc. If high-copper shellfish and nuts aren't balanced with foods that are not only rich in zinc but also low in copper, the consumption of these foods can lead to copper-zinc imbalance.

Whole grains such as whole wheat and rye also can contribute to copper-zinc imbalance. Whole grains typically are listed as good sources of zinc, and they do contain a significant amount. However, because whole grains are rich in insoluble fiber and phytic acid, the zinc they contain is less easily absorbed (or less "bioavailable") than the zinc found in animal protein. Phytic acid is a phosphorus-like compound that binds with zinc and carries it out of the body unused. Insoluble fiber also can interfere with the availability of zinc for absorption. Many people switch from zinc-stripped, white-flour products to whole grains to improve their health, unaware that eating whole grains excessively can actually decrease their zinc status. The more whole grains we eat, the more likely we are to develop zinc deficiency, and (as a result) the more likely we are to experience copper buildup.

Key Drawbacks of Many Natural-Food Diets
- They're disproportionately high in copper and low in zinc.
- They contain excessive phytic acid and insoluble fiber from whole grains, which inhibit the body's absorption of zinc

Celeste had the right idea: a diet based on whole foods is always more nutritious than a diet composed of processed foods. But to prevent zinc deficiency and copper buildup, it's important to avoid an excessive intake of both high-copper foods and phytic acid–containing foods that interfere with zinc absorption. To maintain the necessary delicate balance of copper and zinc in the body, we need to achieve a balance of these minerals in our diet. Unfortunately, vegetarian, macrobiotic, and seafood-based eating plans can disrupt this balance.

Penny, the Lacto-Vegetarian

Penny, a 32-year-old painter, stepped into my office, her face drawn. She told me she had been experiencing severe premenstrual symptoms since a time about five years earlier when she had been under a lot of stress. As a step toward improved general health, as well as to alleviate the premenstrual symptoms, her naturopathic doctor had suggested that she give up red meats and substitute soy foods instead, which she did. Instead of getting better, though, her premenstrual tension had gradually become worse and she had become more tired. She had eventually stopped eating all animal protein except dairy products. Like many American women, Penny was calcium-crazed: she continued to eat dairy foods (even though they didn't seem to agree with her)—and also took 1,000 milligrams of supplemental calcium each day—because she was concerned about the possibility of osteoporosis later in life. (This was in fact a bad plan for preventing osteoporosis, but she had heard too many milk-is-good-for-your-bones commercials.) Also concerned about pesticides, Penny bought only organic foods. A typical daily menu for her looked like this:

- A fruit and yogurt shake with soy protein powder for breakfast
- A veggie-cheese sandwich on a whole-wheat tortilla for lunch
- Veggie sticks and a yogurt dip for snack
- Tofu-veggie-cheese lasagna with a salad for dinner
- A health-food-brand organic chocolate bar or organic ice cream for dessert

THE TROUBLE WITH LACTO-VEGETARIAN DIETS

Penny ate a lacto-vegetarian diet—that is, she emphasized whole grains and soy products in combination with dairy products such as cheese and ice cream. This combination, in my experience, is a common contributor to the development of copper overload. Whole grains, as mentioned previously, contain zinc-inhibiting phytic acid; so too do soy protein foods. Phytic acid significantly reduces zinc absorption, and this effect is made worse by excess calcium in the diet. Research has shown that high calcium intake in the presence of high phytic acid intake (from breads, cereals, and soybeans) has a synergistic effect in decreasing zinc absorption. This means that zinc deficiency is far more likely to occur when whole grains and soy foods are eaten in combination with dairy foods (or when they're taken with high intakes of supplemental calcium).

The combination of whole grains, soy foods, and dairy products can contribute to copper overload in another way. The high calcium content of dairy foods tends to slow the metabolism, as does the high fat content of many dairy foods (such as cheese and ice cream). The slower an individual's metabolism, the less effective the body is at eliminating excess copper, regardless of the person's copper intake. This means that when high-copper, whole-wheat products and soy foods are combined with high-calcium, high-fat cheese, the stage is set for the development (or exacerbation) of copper overload.

Key Drawbacks of Lacto-Vegetarian Diets
- They're high in calcium and sometimes in fat, both of which slow metabolism and increase the likelihood of copper overload.
- They're high in phytic acid (from whole grains and soy foods), which significantly inhibits zinc absorption.

Ironically, individuals with copper imbalance tend to gravitate toward dairy foods: because the excess copper in their systems causes them to feel nervous, they crave the temporary relaxation that the high calcium in dairy foods induces. However, eating these foods frequently worsens their problem by slowing metabolism. When they eat a lot of high-calcium dairy foods together with phytic acid–rich grains and soy products, they further increase their chances of copper overload, because this combination of foods dramatically decreases the body's absorption of copper-antagonistic zinc.

Like many Americans, Penny didn't know anything about the importance of zinc and copper—and a proper balance between the two—for health and energy. She gave up eating zinc-rich meats in favor of high-copper soy foods in large part because she experienced premenstrual syndrome (PMS), and yet PMS is strongly tied to copper-zinc imbalance in the tissues (see Chapter 6). She believed that calcium was all that was needed for healthy bones, and yet the proper balance between zinc and copper plays a critical role as well. To help alleviate her premenstrual symptoms and to protect her energy and bone health, Penny would have been better off deemphasizing both high-calcium dairy foods and high-copper whole grains and soy foods—and adding some zinc-rich meats to her diet.

Dee, the Vegan

Dee, a 44-year-old librarian, sought my advice because she was often tired and depressed and had cold hands and cold feet. She also complained that her skin was excessively dry and her hair was lifeless. Dee told me she had stopped eating animal protein seven years earlier, at first because she lost her taste for it and later because not eating meat became a philosophical issue for her. A typical menu for her included the following:

- A whole-wheat bagel and fruit juice for breakfast
- Bean soup and a salad for lunch
- Whole-grain crackers spread with nut butter for snack
- Tofu/veggie stir-fry for dinner

THE TROUBLE WITH VEGAN DIETS

Vegan diets—those without animal protein of any kind, not even that found in dairy foods—increase the likelihood of copper buildup and/or copper-zinc imbalance, because they differ from well-balanced mixed diets in several key ways. First, they're lower in protein, which, you'll recall, helps with both copper transport and copper detoxification. Second, what protein they do contain—vegetable protein—is of lower quality than animal protein because (1) it's not as digestible, since the fiber within plants inhibits the absorption of amino acids (the building blocks of protein that we obtain from our diet), and (2) it's low or entirely lacking in one or more of those essential amino acids. Most grains, for example, lack the amino acids lysine and threonine, while beans lack methionine. Chosen well, however, the amino acids these foods contain can complement each other to supply good-quality protein. Some vegans are aware of this protein issue and eat a wide variety of legumes, grains, nuts, and seeds over the course of the day to try to meet their protein needs. However, many individuals turn to veganism without knowing anything about the nature of vegetable protein. Thinking that they're eating wisely, they consume a limited range of foods—say, a bagel and fruit for breakfast, a salad for lunch, and pasta for dinner—and fail to get all the amino acids required. As a consequence, they end up deficient in the protein they need for copper utilization and detoxification.

Vegans like Dee who are knowledgeable about the need for a variety of different plant-based protein sources in their diet still are prone to copper buildup. That's because all vegetable protein sources—soy products, beans, whole grains, nuts, and seeds—are high in copper.

Exacerbating the problem, they're also lower in zinc than animal protein sources. As a result, when vegetable protein sources are used in combination to provide a better-quality (more "complete") protein, copper levels get way out of balance with zinc levels. Thus even vegans who manage to obtain adequate protein are still susceptible to copper toxicity. Tissue mineral experts have known for years that copper toxicity is statistically more common in vegetarians than in nonvegetarians. Exaggerated levels of copper in the diet, low levels of zinc (or zinc absorption), and low protein intake all help to explain this phenomenon.

Key Drawbacks of Vegan Diets
- They're low in protein, which is needed for copper utilization and detoxification.
- They're disproportionately high in copper and low in zinc.

Dee had done her homework on protein, but she didn't realize how her copper-rich diet was undermining her health. To improve her low moods and raise her energy, she needed to take steps to promote better copper-zinc balance in her diet by adding zinc-rich foods such as pumpkin seeds and eggs, taking plant-based digestive enzymes to help improve her digestion of protein, and supplementing her diet with zinc.

Jan, the Overdieter

Jan, a 19-year-old college student, came to see me only because her mother insisted. She looked extremely gaunt, frail, and tired, and her mother, who sat in on the appointment, said Jan was almost always sick with the latest bug. Like many young women, Jan had been concerned about her weight ever since puberty, and she had a history of going on and off crash weight-loss diets. At eighteen she had left home to go off to college and had begun drinking alcohol—often way too much alcohol—as a way to fit in and overcome her shyness at parties put on by college fraternities. On her own for the first time in her life, Jan had found herself eating more irregularly than she had when her mother had fixed the meals at home; and with the pressure of college exams, she had been under a lot more stress. When Jan and her mother visited me, Jan reported that she had lost weight several months earlier on a low-calorie fruit-juice diet. Even though Jan had gone off the diet in the meantime, she didn't have an appetite any longer; she just picked at her food. On a good day, her mother said, Jan would have some fruit for breakfast, a salad for lunch, and a bowl of soup for dinner.

THE TROUBLE WITH OVERDIETING

Unfortunately, there's a lot of bad advice circulating about how to lose weight effectively. It's not uncommon to find people like Jan starving themselves on weight-loss diets that are low in protein, calories, and zinc. Going too long without food or eating too little protein or calories causes the body to believe it's starving. It then acts accordingly, conserving energy and slowing the metabolism. This can lead to copper toxicity, because the more sluggish the metabolism becomes, the less effective the body is at detoxifying excess copper. Even after people go off crash diets, their metabolism often stays slow, increasing the likelihood of copper overload in the future.

Key Drawbacks of Crash Weight-Loss Diets
- They're low in protein and calories, a combination that causes metabolism and copper detoxification to become sluggish.
- They're low in zinc, which can lead to a deficiency in that nutrient, causing lack of taste and appetite for food.

People who follow low-calorie, high-carbohydrate, and vegetarian diets to lose weight avoid the richest sources of zinc, which include red meats, poultry, and eggs. Their zinc levels thus plummet along with their weight, leading to long-range consequences. One of zinc's key functions is in the appetite-control center in the brain. When zinc levels dwindle, appetite fails and the senses of smell and taste diminish. As a result of this loss of taste and appetite, some dieters—Jan among them—find it almost impossible to resume normal eating habits after they've reached their intended weight goal. Zinc deficiency is strongly linked to eating disorders, and many women who have a history of dieting seem to be in what I believe is a "pre-anorexic" state. They eat like birds yet simply aren't hungry. A vicious cycle then develops: the more their appetite diminishes, the less food they eat. The less food they eat, the more their metabolism slows. And the more their metabolism slows, the more readily copper accumulates.

Many people would be surprised to learn that Jan would've experienced better health and energy—and longer-lasting weight loss (because what she lost would've been fat, not muscle)—by eating a higher-calorie diet containing foods high in zinc-rich animal protein, such as eggs, poultry, and meats. This type of diet keeps the metabolism stronger so that it can burn fat more effectively and eliminate copper properly. To improve her appetite so that she could begin to eat this type of diet, Jan, like Dee, needed to take regular zinc supplements, along with digestive enzymes to help her digestion and absorption of protein.

THE GROWING PROBLEM OF ZINC DEFICIENCY

Many dietary factors contribute to copper overload, but the biggest one by far, in my opinion, is zinc deficiency. The simple truth is it's much more difficult for us to meet our zinc needs through diet than it was for our ancestors.

Lack of Zinc in Our Soil

Acid rain and aggressive agricultural practices developed during this century have severely depleted the zinc in our soil, and therefore in our diet. Plants absorb minerals from the soil into their complex structures; people then consume the minerals either directly (from fruits and vegetables) or indirectly (via plant-fed poultry and livestock). The link is clear and direct: when our soil is deficient in zinc, the plants and animals we eat are deficient too. Researchers working for the U.S. Department of Agriculture in the 1970s found that the soil in at least thirty states was severely lacking in zinc, and it's believed that the deficit is even more widespread today. Although plant foods such as fruits and vegetables have never been major sources of dietary zinc, they used to provide small but steady amounts—much more than they now supply.

Food Processing

Just as modern agricultural practices have depleted zinc in our foods, so too have modern food-processing techniques. The depletion of zinc in the milling of grains has already been discussed, but other processing and preserving techniques also cause zinc to be lost. Canned beans, for example, lose 60 percent of the zinc contained in fresh beans, canned tomatoes 45 percent, and canned spinach 40 percent. Americans in particular like foods that are quick and ready-to-eat, but they pay a price for eating processed convenience foods. That price includes a growing zinc deficiency.

Zinc-Zappers

Many factors act as zinc-zappers, further compounding the problem of lack of zinc in our diet. These include:

Stress
Coffee
Alcohol
Sugar
A high-carbohydrate diet
Some diuretics and antacids
Cortisone

In addition, surgery, burns, injury, weight loss, illness, oral contraceptives, and pregnancy all cause dramatic increases in our need for zinc. And the problem is hereditary: pregnant women who are deficient in zinc can transmit this imbalance to their children through the placenta. This means that many children in the next generation may be born with zinc deficiency.

Because of all these factors, the late Carl C. Pfeiffer, Ph.D., M.D.—a brilliant researcher and the founder of Princeton BioCenter in Skillman, New Jersey—maintained that every American in this day and age is borderline deficient in zinc. Survey data indicate that average zinc intake ranges from 47 to 67 percent of the recommended daily allowance of 15 milligrams a day for men, 12 milligrams a day for women. This indicates at least a marginal zinc deficiency. Based on my experience, however, I've concluded that many women don't consume even this inadequate amount of zinc.

It's not politically correct to say this, but the best way to obtain an adequate amount of zinc through diet is by eating small, consistent amounts of animal protein—especially red meats, eggs, and poultry.

Many women especially have cut down on or completely eliminated these foods from their diet, favoring instead foods that are high in carbohydrates. But as we have seen, the amount of protein in our diet influences how well the body absorbs and retains zinc: low-protein, high-carbohydrate diets lower zinc levels, while high-protein, moderate-carbohydrate diets increase zinc status. This means that the string of "light" diets so popular today—from low-fat, high-carbohydrate, to macrobiotic, to vegetarian, to crash weight-loss diets—all worsen the zinc deficiency problem, setting the stage for copper overload to develop.

FOOD FOR THOUGHT ABOUT "LIGHT" DIETS

"Light" diets have become popular in recent years because most of us have heard—and believed—a lot of erroneous information describing fat and animal protein as fattening and disease-promoting. We've been told that if we avoid fat and animal protein and load up on carbohydrates, we'll be energetic, thin, and healthy enough to ward off killer diseases such as heart disease and diabetes. Many people have taken this advice to heart and adopted a low-fat, high-carbohydrate diet, only to find that this diet doesn't do what it's been advertised to do. In the last several decades, Americans as a whole have cut their fat intake, decreased their red meat consumption, and dramatically increased their intake of carbohydrates just as has been recommended, yet levels of obesity have skyrocketed, heart disease rates haven't improved, and diabetes rates have tripled. There's a simple reason for this: high levels of carbohydrates in the diet raise levels of insulin (a blood sugar–balancing hormone), and high insulin levels promote obesity, diabetes, and heart disease.

As I've discussed, high-carbohydrate plant-based diets also promote copper toxicity—something very few medical practitioners know about. Since copper overload goes hand in hand with fatigue and other health problems, it isn't any wonder that many of us who eat "light" find ourselves feeling lousy. We're following the wrong diet—a diet that's contributing to our health problems and lack of energy.

Point to Ponder #1: If you began eating a high-carbohydrate diet for health reasons but now find yourself more tired, emotional, anxious, or susceptible to sickness, it's time to reevaluate just how healthy the "light" diet you're following really is. If you have copper toxicity (or are prone to it), you need to understand that a high-carbohydrate diet simply isn't good for you.

Many people switch to a lighter diet because red meats and other types of animal protein feel "heavy" in their system. Ironically, this feeling can develop from copper excess or zinc deficiency (or adrenal insufficiency, which you'll learn about in Chapter 5). Individuals with copper-zinc imbalance have trouble digesting and absorbing fat and protein in particular, so they often opt for diets that avoid foods rich in these nutrients. At first it might be only red meat that feels like a brick in their digestive tract, so they avoid it. Then, as their zinc deficiency or copper imbalance gradually worsens, they begin having trouble digesting other types of animal protein and usually eliminate them one by one—first poultry, then fish, then eggs and dairy products, on down the line. Yet the more an individual with copper imbalance eats a low-protein, high-carbohydrate diet, the more his or her metabolism will slow; then, as a consequence, the copper overload will worsen and digestion will further decline.

Point to Ponder #2: If you have trouble digesting meat or find yourself attracted to low-fat, high-carbohydrate diets, you should suspect a copper-zinc imbalance.

Many of my clients who have been vegetarians or high-carbohydrate eaters at one time have told me that they turned to these diets primarily because they found meat not agreeing with them. Looking at this issue in retrospect, my clients have said that their difficulty digesting meat began shortly after they started feeling exhausted and experiencing other typical copper overload symptoms.

Point to Ponder #3: If you became a vegetarian for philosophical rather than dietary motives, you need to reevaluate your reasoning.

Many individuals try a plant-based (or mostly plant-based) diet because they think it's an environmentally and socially conscious thing to do. This was certainly a factor for me when I became a vegetarian in college in the early 1970s. I've always considered myself spiritually conscious, concerned about the health of the planet and the welfare of animals: I liked the idea of not eating animal protein, and all the information I read about vegetarianism back in college seemed to support my choice to avoid meat. But the fact is human beings evolved on animal protein, and it's virtually impossible to obtain adequate amounts of dietary zinc any other way. Beef, for example, has a fourfold greater bioavailability of zinc than do high-fiber cereals. Pronounced zinc deficiency has been known to occur in populations whose zinc intake is far in excess of the National Academy of Sciences recommended amount but is derived exclusively from vegetable sources. I didn't have access to this information when I was in college, so I strictly followed a plant-based diet. After about a year on that vegan diet, however, I was noticeably weak and constantly craved sweets for quick energy, my skin was covered with acne, and my hair was falling out. My body was telling me in no uncertain terms that it was starving for zinc! People who avoid meat certainly can take zinc supplements, and I do recommend them. But while supplemental zinc can be helpful, it's never absorbed into the body as well as the zinc in animal protein is.

Point to Ponder #3: If you've been puzzled by a lack of energy and vitality lately, you should evaluate your diet. In my experience, a diet that's low in zinc, low in protein, or high in copper is almost always a factor in these symptoms.

Chapter Four

Copper Culprits and Environmental Factors That Can Contribute to Fatigue

Various environmental factors unique to our age either con-tribute excessive amounts of copper to the body or interfere with the body's ability to excrete copper. From the water we drink to the plethora of chemicals we're exposed to, many culprits make us much more susceptible to copper overload and the fatigue that accompanies it than our ancestors were.

A SURVEY OF ENVIRONMENTAL COPPER

Copper is ubiquitous in our environment, found in everything from wiring to pipes to fungicides. It's common, therefore, for many of us to get external exposure to copper on a regular or even frequent basis. Here's a quick rundown of some of the most common environmental sources:

Water
Water is the most important human nutrient besides oxygen, but these days we need to be very careful about our water supply: it can

contain unhealthy levels of copper for a variety of reasons. Some areas of the country simply have high amounts of naturally occurring copper in their water supply, while many municipal water companies add copper sulfate to the water supply to kill algae and fungi. Copper water pipes have been in widespread use in U.S. homes for the last several decades, and they can leach copper into the water supply if the water is extremely acidic or alkaline or if it has a very low total dissolved solid content (as purified or distilled water does). Copper tubing is used in many water coolers and ice-makers in refrigerators as well, so water that sits in these units sometimes contains very high levels of copper.

Dental Materials
Dental fillings—especially those made of the newer silver amalgams and certain gold alloys—are a surprising contributor to copper overload. Many of my clients, aware that the mercury found in older fillings is toxic, switched to the newer compounds, not knowing that doing so was essentially jumping from the fire into the frying pan. Mercury amalgams are undesirable for a variety of reasons, of course—not the least of which is that mercury interferes with normal liver function and with copper excretion. But many of the newer silver amalgams and some gold alloys contain significant amounts of copper. They release almost imperceptible—but steady and sustained—levels of this unbound toxin into the system over their many years of service. The best bet for fillings at this point appears to be a nonreactive composite that's metal-free.

Pesticides and Other Chemicals
Chemicals abound in our society, contributing to copper overload and fatigue in both direct and indirect ways. Some chemicals, such as copper sulfate—a fungicide used in swimming pools and on produce—directly increase the body's copper burden. Other chemicals, those known as xenoestrogens, are found in pesticides, plastics, household cleaners, and automobile exhaust. Because these xenoestrogens have an estrogen-like molecular structure, they can cause a buildup of estrogen in the body, thereby inhibiting the body's ability to eliminate copper. Other chemicals—though they aren't direct sources of copper or estrogen—tax the liver's ability to eliminate toxins, including excess copper.

Other Sources
Other minor sources of environmental copper contribute to our copper burden. Copper tea kettles and other copper cookware, for example, can be a source of toxicity if used frequently over a period of time. Copper cookware can be especially hazardous to health when acidic foods (such as those containing vinegar) come in contact with it.

Copper also is added to many nutrient supplements, especially prenatal vitamins, sometimes in significant amounts. The extra copper can be harmful to people prone to copper overload—in other words, those who can't eliminate excess copper properly. People who work directly with copper—such as plumbers, welders, machinists, jewelry makers, and artists—are at particular risk for copper toxicity.

COMMONLY USED DRUGS AS COPPER CULPRITS

Many common drugs, nonprescription as well as prescription, increase a person's likelihood of developing copper overload. Cortisone, Tagamet, Zantac, antacids, and many diuretics, for example, significantly impair zinc absorption. (Zinc deficiency, as mentioned earlier, is one of the most common contributors to copper excess.) Another substance that we don't think of as a drug—alcohol— also precipitates zinc deficiency by flushing zinc out of the system. Beer and certain other types of alcohol are double trouble, because they're also high in copper.

Any medications that interfere with liver or gallbladder function elevate copper, because excess copper is normally excreted through bile. Common drugs that can adversely affect liver or gallbladder function include some sedatives, tranquilizers, and psychotropic medications, as well as estrogen medications.

The Birth Control Pill and Other Estrogen Medications
Widespread use of estrogen medications such as the birth control pill is one of the main reasons for the prevalence of copper overload today, according to many copper overload experts. Though "the pill" has been prescribed liberally for the past four decades, it's known to make liver and gallbladder function sluggish and to increase copper levels.

Some women who have low copper levels feel better when they start taking the pill, because the estrogen contained in the pill elevates their copper. If a woman stays on the pill long enough, however, copper levels can rise past normal, leading to the development of copper overload. Use of the pill or estrogen replacement therapy can be particularly problematic for women who have high estrogen levels to begin with or who are prone to copper overload because of a slow metabolism or other factors. The more these women use estrogen medications, the more copper-toxic they can become.

Copper IUDs

Copper intrauterine devices (IUDs) are a direct source of consistent exposure to dangerous levels of copper. The body can absorb several hundred milligrams of copper from a copper IUD, and these high levels in the uterus greatly increase the likelihood of liver dysfunction and pelvic inflammatory disease.

HEREDITY AS A FACTOR IN COPPER OVERLOAD

According to copper overload expert Dr. Lawrence Wilson, of Prescott, Arizona, copper-toxic women can unknowingly pass a copper excess on to their unborn children. As a result, many children come into the world with copper overload or copper-zinc imbalance. Problems that can result in children from congenital copper imbalance include learning and behavior difficulties, immune system weaknesses, allergies, and recurring infections.

If copper toxicity is passed on from generation to generation, copper-related health problems are likely to become worse. Rick Malter, Ph.D., a psychologist with the Malter Institute for Natural Development in Hoffman Estates, Illinois, who's been treating copper-related mental and emotional health problems for 18 years, explains this phenomenon (institute reference sheet, 1984):

> A female child born to a mother who has a copper excess will begin life with a higher copper level then her mother began life. Throughout her developing years, such a female child is likely to accumulate more and more copper in her tissues, especially during pre-adolescence and adolescence when her own estrogen produc-

tion increases. She is likely to give birth to children who will absorb higher amounts of copper than she absorbed *in utero*. In each succeeding generation, this cycle is likely to repeat itself resulting in more and more children born with significant copper excess.

WHEN OUR COPPER LOAD IS TOO GREAT

Each of the factors listed in this chapter can contribute to copper overload. Although the body is designed to eliminate a certain amount of excess copper, when factors that increase our copper burden accumulate, they can cause a total load that's simply too much for the body to cope with; illness then results. To understand how copper overload can gradually develop and escalate because of many environmental factors, consider the story of Jane Ayres, M.A., L.M.H.C., a psychotherapist and instructor in psychology at the University of Massachusetts.

Jane

Jane had experienced symptoms such as an overactive mind, a tired body, and mild depression and anxiety for about a decade, but like most women she had no idea copper overload was involved. Unaware of the many contributors to copper overload in our environment, she was exposed to numerous factors that caused her condition to escalate. First, the water in her town had unusually high naturally occurring copper levels, registering in the 90th percentile for copper. (In other words, only 10 percent of water supplies have more copper.) Even without that formal evaluation, though, there was evidence of the culprit: all her sinks and tubs had blue-green staining, which is a telltale sign of high copper in the water. "I unfortunately didn't know that and drank that water for four years," Jane recalls. "Even after I switched to drinking spring water, I still continued to bathe in that high-copper water, not knowing that copper could be absorbed through the skin."[1]

[1] *Unless otherwise noted, quotations in this and all subsequent case studies are from interviews conducted by the author either in person, by phone, or in writing.*

For 11 years, Jane also took birth control pills, which undoubtedly increased her copper burden. "And I did another thing that in retrospect was bad," Jane recounts. "I had some skin problems when I was younger, so I took antibiotics literally like they were candy for about ten years. The antibiotics seemed to clear up my face and I was very happy about that, but I didn't realize that they were also causing inhibition of the excretion of the copper." Like many individuals who have copper overload, Jane also found herself attracted to high-copper foods such as shellfish and nuts, and ate these foods repetitively.

The cumulative load of all the copper culprits in Jane's life led to a worsening of her health. In 1990 Jane began dropping things, started to feel even more tired than usual, and developed overall muscle weakness and a rag-doll feeling. She eventually learned that her symptoms were due to a type of neuropathy (nerve dysfunction) possibly triggered by the extremely high levels of copper both in her blood and in her tissues.

Jane had a severe case of copper overload, but there's a bright ending to her story. After she learned about copper overload, she began taking some key copper-lowering nutrient supplements (which you'll learn more about in Chapter 10) and changed her diet—and the copper levels in her blood came down quickly. "Within four weeks, I was 85 percent better. I was absolutely amazed," Jane says. Her tissue copper levels took longer to come down, but as they did her health improved by leaps and bounds. "The discovery of that high copper was a major turning point in my life," Jane explains. "I'm still amazed at how one mineral can affect you so dramatically, when it's in toxic amounts—and how much healthier I am now than I used to be."

Jane's experience of recurrent exposure to copper contributors is echoed in many homes across the country. Her story shows that water, commonly prescribed drugs, and environmental culprits are contributors to copper overload that we must take seriously to safeguard our health and energy.

Chapter Five

Stress, Burnout, and Blood Sugar Imbalance

Of all the contributors to copper-induced fatigue, excessive stress is the most important. Unfortunately, as we all know, it's also one of the toughest to beat. Even if we eat a diet that balances copper and zinc and we avoid external sources of copper, we still can develop copper overload and the fatigue that comes with it if we're faced with too much stress.

THE STRESS CONNECTION TO HIGH COPPER AND LOW ZINC

The body loses zinc quickly under stress. In fact, zinc comes pouring out of the urine as part of the natural fight-or-flight response. Anything we perceive as threatening to our physical or emotional health—that is, any *stressor*—causes us distress. The more stressors we experience, the more our zinc levels drop. I probably don't need to remind you of the common stressors, but here goes:

COMMON STRESSORS

Unresolved negative emotions: fear, worry, anger, sadness, guilt, or grief
Lack of sleep

Undereating
Excessive intake of sugar or stimulants
Physical injury
Surgery
Overwork
Overexercise
Exposure to temperature extremes
Exposure to chemical toxins

In our modern lives—replete with pressures from work and family, on top of the pressures most of us put on ourselves—we often encounter both major stressors and a constant bombardment of minor stressors that cause zinc levels to plummet. Zinc and copper compete for absorption, as I've noted, so when levels of zinc in the body drop, copper climbs, replacing zinc in the tissues.

THE ADRENAL CONNECTION TO COPPER IMBALANCE

In addition to depleting zinc, excessive stress can also weaken the functioning of our adrenal glands. The "stress glands" constantly respond to the stressors we encounter in our daily lives, producing hormones that help balance blood sugar. Since blood sugar is the fuel that virtually all body cells (especially brain cells) require for energy, the adrenals in effect make sure we have the right amount of fuel to meet our varying demands for energy. When we run into stressful situations, we require more energy to cope, so the adrenals kick in with the extra get-up-and-go we need. Few of us appreciate how many stressors the adrenals respond to every day; they're mighty workhorses. But, like everything else, they have a limited supply of energy. If we have an excessive stress load and can't creatively cope with the stress we can't avoid, the adrenals weaken, no longer producing adequate amounts of stress hormones. This is when copper overload can set in.

According to Paul C. Eck, a researcher who studied tissue mineral states and their effects on health for 25 years, weak adrenal gland function is the most important physiological cause of copper imbalance. Healthy adrenal activity is required to build proteins, including one called ceruloplasmin, which is the main copper-binding protein in the body. Ceruloplasmin is necessary for the proper transportation and utilization of copper. If the adrenals become weak from too much stress, the liver makes less ceruloplasmin, and unbound copper starts to gather in various tissues and organs.

Healthy adrenals also send signals to the liver to detoxify and excrete excess copper. If adrenal function is diminished, then copper retention rises. The weaker the adrenal glands become, the more metabolism slows, and the more copper tends to accumulate.

The connection between adrenal insufficiency and copper imbalance goes two ways. You might remember from Chapter 2 that copper excess or zinc deficiency also diminishes adrenal gland function. This means that *the more stress we're under, the more likely we are to develop copper excess or zinc deficiency that leads to adrenal insufficiency—and the more likely we are to develop adrenal insufficiency that leads to copper excess or copper-zinc imbalance!* It's not surprising, therefore, that individuals who have copper overload almost always have adrenal insufficiency.

Copper excess or zinc deficiency can cause adrenal insufficiency to escalate into a more advanced stage called *adrenal exhaustion* or *adrenal burnout,* which is characterized by extreme fatigue. This is a situation I see all too often among the many talented professionals I counsel. Unfortunately, adrenal burnout—like copper overload—goes unrecognized by most conventionally trained doctors.

THE MISUNDERSTOOD CONDITION OF ADRENAL BURNOUT

Traditional medicine recognizes only the most extreme form of adrenal burnout: Addison's disease, a potentially life-threatening condition in which the adrenals make no cortisol hormones. However, there's a wide spectrum of diminishing function between healthy adrenals and Addison's disease. A person could feel horrible and have virtually no energy because of poor adrenal function and yet not show any abnormalities on the standard adrenal function test.

Many alternative-minded health professionals have been aware of the adrenal continuum for many years and now use more sophisticated tests to determine varying degrees of diminished adrenal activity. Tissue mineral analysis, for example, is one good way to determine subclinical adrenal insufficiency. Another test, called the adrenal stress index, measures salivary levels of the adrenal hormones dehy-droepiandrosterone (DHEA) and cortisol several times throughout the day; low levels of these hormones indicate adrenal burnout. (For information on how you can have salivary levels of your adrenal hormones measured, see the Resources section in the back of the book.)

Leonid Wilson, M.D., a holistic practitioner from Burlington, Massachusetts, uses both tests in his practice and has found that copper overload and adrenal burnout go hand in hand. Dr. Wilson told me, "The story [with many people who have copper overload] is that they have been pushing, pushing, pushing themselves—or not coping well with the stresses in their lives." He said, "This progressively reduces adrenal reserves, leading to adrenal burnout and chronic fatigue."

The adrenals produce hormones that perform countless functions in the body in their effort to keep us healthy. When the adrenals become exhausted, hormone production diminishes and numerous symptoms can develop.

COMMON SYMPTOMS OF ADRENAL BURNOUT

Chronic fatigue or exhaustion
Cravings for sweets due to the need for quick energy
Cravings for salt due to low sodium levels
Low blood pressure
Attraction to stimulants because of extreme fatigue
The feeling of being overwhelmed by stress
Food or environmental allergies
Low immune function
Symptoms of hypoglycemia or diabetes
Distaste for meat protein due to impaired digestion
Premenstrual symptoms or menopausal difficulties

The fatigue experienced by those with copper overload and adrenal burnout differs from simple fatigue. Many of us have experienced the kind of fatigue that results from being overworked or not getting enough sleep. This sensation goes away when we rest for a bit, get caught up on our sleep, or take a vacation. But burnout, as the term suggests, is more than that: the adrenals literally are exhausted, so the body is tired all the time. This type of fatigue can't be corrected by simple rest or a vacation. Because the adrenals are underfunction-ing, they simply aren't able to give the body the energy it needs to rise to the challenge of stressful situations. The fatigue can be so over-whelming for individuals with adrenal burnout that they become compulsive about anything that gives them a lift. They feel the need for frequent coffee to get (and keep) going, for example, or they turn to "natural" herbal stimulants for quick charges of pep. They usually also crave sugar to provide the quick energy they're lacking.

THE BLOOD SUGAR BLUES

Lack of energy and cravings for sugar are common in those with adrenal burnout and copper overload, because much of the fatigue suffered by these individuals is brought on by faulty blood sugar reg-ulation. Balanced blood sugar is of utmost importance to the body. If blood sugar drops too low, the body perceives this as a major stress: the muscles and brain sense that they're running out of fuel for energy. The adrenals normally respond to this situation by releasing the stress hormones adrenaline and cortisol, which signal the liver to convert protein to sugar (a process known as *gluconeogenesis*), thus raising blood sugar to a higher, steady level. When the adrenals are burned out, however, they produce such low amounts of these hor-mones that they aren't able to properly convey messages to the liver. Hypoglycemia (that is, low blood sugar)—a condition that causes the distressing symptoms listed below—then results.

COMMON SYMPTOMS OF HYPOGLYCEMIA

Fatigue or sleepiness
Headaches
Depression
Irritability
Cravings for sugar
Mood swings
Weakness
Poor concentration
Poor memory
Dizziness, lightheadedness

Hypoglycemia also can develop when liver function isn't up to par. If the liver is burdened with too many toxins, too much stored copper, or a poor copper-to-zinc ratio, the function of the liver can become so sluggish that it's unable to perform adequate gluconeogenesis. This means that blood sugar levels stay low, depriving brain and muscles of the fuel they need for proper energy and stamina.

Steady blood sugar levels for sustained energy also depend upon adequate levels of zinc. This mineral is needed for the production and secretion of hydrochloric acid in the stomach and pancreatic enzymes in the pancreas. If a zinc deficiency or copper excess exists, protein digestion and assimilation are impaired, and the liver lacks an adequate supply of the amino acids (protein constituents) that it converts to blood sugar. Without sufficient amounts of amino acids for the liver to use, blood sugar levels stay low, resulting in physical and mental fatigue.

Individuals with copper-zinc imbalance can develop another type of blood sugar imbalance: high blood sugar, or diabetes. Zinc is needed to make, secrete, and store the hormone insulin and to extend the action of that hormone. Insulin, secreted from the pancreas after carbohydrates are eaten, lowers sugar levels in the blood and drives sugar into the cells, where it can be used as fuel for energy. If zinc deficiency, copper excess, or a poor copper-to-zinc ratio exists, the pancreas can't secrete adequate amounts of insulin and/or the insulin that *is* released can't work as effectively as it should. When either of these situations occurs, blood sugar levels remain elevated, causing diabetes. Without adequate insulin to drive sugar into the cells, the cells are in effect starved for the fuel they need, and lack of energy ensues.

This all may seem a bit complicated, and indeed it is! I admit that the various connections between copper overload and blood sugar regulation can be difficult to follow, because blood sugar regulation involves an intricate system of checks and balances. Here are the main points you need to understand:

• Balanced blood sugar levels for sustained energy require optimal functioning of the adrenals, the pancreas, and the liver. Copper overload or zinc deficiency can adversely affect any one of these organs, leading to blood sugar fluctuations associated with fatigue.

- Adrenal burnout is a major cause of fatigue in and of itself, and it can lead to copper overload, which also causes exhaustion. The adrenals typically become exhausted from too much stress, from zinc deficiency, or from copper buildup.
- When the adrenals become exhausted, protein synthesis—specifically, production of copper-binding ceruloplasmin—diminishes, and liver detoxification slows. Both of these factors contribute to copper buildup and fatigue.

The bottom line is that stress, adrenal exhaustion, blood sugar imbalance, and copper overload often are interconnected. Linda Lizotte, R.D., C.D.N.—a nutritionist in private practice in Trumbull, Connecticut—is one of the many people who've learned this lesson firsthand. Here's her story.

Linda

In 1990, about five months after her first child was born, Linda began experiencing severe exhaustion, especially in the afternoon; frequent severe bruising; and sugar cravings, irritability, headaches, and difficulty concentrating when she went too long without food. "As a nutritionist, I was frustrated because I knew the symptoms I was experiencing were indicative of hypoglycemia, and I tried to follow the standard advice to eat meals with protein more often; but even when I did, my symptoms weren't getting a lot better," she recalls. "I also wondered why these symptoms had developed all of a sudden and why they were so severe."

While she was searching for answers, she stumbled upon a clue that would help her understand that copper overload and adrenal burnout were the underlying causes of the symptoms she experienced. Her hair had become what she calls "dull, flat, and lifeless," so she went to a hair salon to get a permanent wave. To her surprise, the perm didn't take. The people at the hair salon were surprised as well; they didn't know what to make of it. Linda repeated the perm four times, but it never took. Soon after her fourth attempt, Linda found out why.

"I went to a lecture [on tissue mineral analysis], and the speaker mentioned in passing that high copper levels can cause an inability of the hair to perm. I did a double-take, and my mouth dropped open!" she recalls. "He also pointed out that during pregnancy, estrogen levels rise, and when estrogen goes up in the body, copper goes up too." All this seemed to fit Linda's experience perfectly, so shortly after the lecture, Linda had a tissue mineral analysis performed. The results, as you might expect, showed copper levels way off the charts: a normal copper level is 2.5 milligrams per one hundred grams of hair, but Linda's level was 57!

What caused Linda's high copper levels? Pregnancy contributed to her problem, but the main cause, according to Linda, was adrenal burnout brought on by too much stress. "In the course of just a few years, I planned a wedding, got married, started a nutritional counseling business of my own, put in many 12-hour work days, often missed lunch because I was so busy working, moved twice, and had my first baby," says Linda, who sounds tired just recounting her experience. "I didn't really think too much about it, but I definitely was burning the candle at both ends."

After learning about the stress/adrenal connection to copper overload, Linda made the changes that were necessary to turn her health around. She began scheduling a break for lunch every day, made sure she got more sleep, learned to say no to extra projects she didn't *have* to do, and took more time for relaxation generally. She also took an adrenal-supportive nutrient supplement to promote better adrenal function and a copper-lowering supplement to reverse the copper overload in her tissues. (You'll learn more about these helpful nutrient supplements in Chapter 10). And she started eating more protein throughout the day, especially at breakfast.

"One of the things that really helped me was having lunch and dinner for breakfast. What I mean is that I began having nontraditional breakfasts—things like a leftover lamb chop and brown rice in the morning instead of traditional breakfast foods like a bagel or cereal." This gave Linda much more energy throughout the day, and the added protein in her diet boosted her metabolism and helped encourage detoxification of the stored copper. As a result, her copper levels slowly but surely came down, and all the distressing symptoms she'd experienced gradually lessened and one by one disappeared.

Since the time Linda treated herself for copper overload, she's counseled many individuals who have the condition. Although her clients often want to blame their symptoms on high copper in the water or other external factors, most often these factors aren't primary. Based on both Linda's experience and my own, I've concluded that the biggest contributor to copper overload and the fatigue that comes with it is adrenal burnout, a product of too much stress.

Chapter Six

More Than Fatigue: The Copper Connection to Various Health Problems

Fatigue is the most common symptom cited by those with a history of copper overload, but it's certainly not the only one. It generally heads the pack of a conglomeration of disturbing and sometimes baffling health complaints. This chapter will cover the most common copper-related health problems—everything from anxiety to premenstrual syndrome—that people experience along with fatigue.

Before I explain how copper overload can cause these many symptoms, let me tell you a little about how copper overload presented itself in me. Like many people, especially women, I had been bothered by a number of puzzling symptoms during many phases of my life. Back then I had no idea that copper overload was at the root of my problems. Knowing what I now know, however, I believe that I had copper overload as far back as high school.

My Story

For most of my life, I've had sensitive skin. In fact, that's why I became involved with nutrition in the first place. I learned early on that certain foods would trigger a skin breakout. Chocolate, sugary foods of all kinds, nuts, wheat germ, shellfish—even too much fruit or fruit juice!—were off limits for my reactive skin.

In individuals with copper overload, skin problems typically go with the territory, because the skin is an organ of detoxification. When the body's detoxification processes are sluggish, as they usually are in individuals with copper overload, various skin conditions can erupt—quite literally!

I mentioned in Chapter 3 that I had acne when I was in college as a result of my strictly vegan diet. This was both embarrassing and frustrating for me. The blemishes I had took forever to heal, and when they did heal they left a reddish mark. I thought I'd be scarred for life! Acne, as you'll read a little later in this chapter, is frequently associated with zinc deficiency—a condition that, as you well know by now, usually goes hand in hand with copper overload.

In the mid-1980s, I worked at the Pritikin Longevity Center and, like everyone else at the center, ate what I call a "spa-type" diet high in carbohydrates. I'm now convinced that this led to higher copper levels and lower zinc levels in my body. I also had some cavities filled with gold alloys, not knowing that the new gold compound I had chosen was high in copper. Then, in 1988, I went on my first major book tour for my book *Beyond Pritikin* (Bantam, 1988). Although this was an exciting time for me, it also was an incredibly stressful period of my life. I was always on the go—traveling from city to city, grabbing irregular meals when I had the chance, and struggling to sleep in a different hotel room every night.

About this time, I began to have a number of unusual symptoms. First, my hair started to develop an odd orange tint. I didn't know it then, but a hair-color change like that often indicates copper overload. Then I began to feel a real dichotomy between my mind and my body: my mind was always in overdrive, but my body felt tired and unable to keep up. I suffered from many fitful nights of sleep because my mind simply wouldn't shut off, and I found myself feeling more anxious than usual, sometimes downright panicky.

These symptoms were all very confusing to me, because I'd stayed up-to-date on all the latest health information and felt that I was doing almost everything right. This clustering of symptoms peaked just a short while after I'd started to see a pattern of high tissue copper levels in many of my clients (as described in Chapter 1).

One day, while I was thinking about the problems a particular copper-overload client had, I suddenly realized that the answer to my health problems might be right under my nose—*I* might have copper overload too! To satisfy my curiosity, I had a tissue mineral analysis performed. Sure enough, the results came back showing high copper and low zinc levels.

Once I determined the culprit behind my health problems, I took steps to reverse the copper overload. I avoided high-copper foods and made sure I had a steady, consistent supply of zinc in my diet; I took copper-lowering supplements, as well as supplements that supported healthy adrenal and liver function; and I brought some semblance of order to my busy schedule and made more time for myself. I also used myself as a guinea pig, trying a wide variety of supplements and natural remedies, keeping only those that were extremely helpful for both me and my clients. My personal experience helped me fine-tune the copper overload program I'd already begun to develop for my clients—a program you'll read about in Chapters 8 through 11—and I can tell you firsthand it works. Within about six months or so, my copper levels had come down. The more they decreased, the more I felt calm, balanced, and physically energetic.

When I got over the surprise of discovering that I, a nutritionist, could develop copper overload and not know it, I realized how widespread the problem could be. After all, I'd experienced anxiety, insomnia, and a tired body and overactive mind, all of which are very common complaints of women; and I've since learned that many other typical "female" health problems are associated with the condition. The following is a rundown of how copper overload and copper-zinc imbalance can contribute to these various complaints.

ANXIETY, RACING MIND, PANIC ATTACKS, AND INSOMNIA

Zinc is an anti-anxiety mineral. It's not surprising, therefore, that certain of my symptoms—the anxiety, racing mind (inability to stop thoughts), panic attacks, and insomnia—are associated with copper-zinc imbalance. Copper stimulates production of biogenic amines—neurotransmitting substances such as epinephrine, norepinephrine, dopamine, and serotonin—that heighten brain and nervous system activity. Anxiety, racing mind, and insomnia are believed to be caused by imbalances in these neurotransmitters.

Anxiety can have another source as well. As we saw in an earlier chapter, copper excess or zinc deficiency also can diminish activity of the adrenal glands, which help provide the extra energy needed to cope with stress. If the adrenals aren't functioning up to par and we therefore feel overwhelmed by stress, it's understandable that we constantly think about what we have to do, becoming anxious or even panic-stricken, and have trouble sleeping because of it.

Anxiety and panic states also can result from an excessive secretion of adrenaline from the adrenals—a stress response when the blood sugar drops too low. Hypoglycemia, you may remember, can be caused by both copper overload and adrenal dysfunction.

ROLLER-COASTER EMOTIONS

Exaggerated emotional responses—both highs and lows—are frequently experienced by individuals who have copper overload. When the liver becomes overburdened with copper, the body begins to store the excess amounts in other organs, especially the brain. Copper stimulates the diencephalon, which is considered the "old" or "emotional" brain. High levels of copper can therefore cause intense emotional reactions. Zinc, on the other hand, stimulates the cortex, or "new" brain, which overlays the old brain and tends to tone down its activity. Normal zinc levels encourage calmness and equanimity in the face of stress.

The late Carl Pfeiffer taught an entire generation of nutritionally oriented psychiatrists that many psychological problems, ranging from depression to schizophrenia, can be caused by high copper levels. The types of emotional states experienced by those with copper overload or copper-zinc imbalance vary according to the individual, the degree of mineral imbalance, and the organs and tissues affected. Depression, for example, can result when high copper levels slow down the functioning of the thyroid gland, causing low energy. Depression is also a common side effect of oral contraceptives, which cause copper levels to rise in the body. Emotional hyperactivity, on the other hand, can occur when high copper levels affect the diencephalon. This imbalance arises quite often during stressful situations, because zinc levels drop and copper levels rise.

Often individuals with copper overload alternate between emotional highs and lows, depending on such factors as how much stress they're experiencing, what they've recently eaten, what medications they're taking, and (in the case of women) what phase of the menstrual cycle they're in. Psychologist Rick Malter says he sees many cases of what he calls "pseudo–bipolar disorder." While most mental health professionals label this variant of true bipolar disorder a manic-depressive condition, Malter identifies it as a copper toxicity problem. He estimates that 70 to 80 percent of the clients he sees in his practice for various emotional and psychological problems have copper overload.

SKIN PROBLEMS

Copper overload and copper-zinc imbalance are related to a wide variety of skin problems, because both copper and zinc play important roles in the health of the skin. Copper helps to form pigment in the skin, for example, so excess copper can lead to dark areas of pigmentation, especially on the face. (This condition is most often seen in women with high estrogen levels.)

Zinc is a vital nutrient for the healing of bruises and wounds and for helping to prevent acne. Zinc deficiency, which as we've seen often occurs in conjunction with copper overload, has been found in patients with skin blemishes, psoriasis, rashes, and slow wound healing.

In copper overload, the skin is often affected, because the skin— like the liver—is an organ of detoxification, as I noted earlier. If the liver isn't doing a good job of eliminating toxic materials from the body—as is usually the case in copper overload—additional toxins come out through the skin, decreasing skin quality and increasing the likelihood of acne and rashes.

Copper overload also can cause a lack of essential fatty acids in the body. These are the good fats needed for soft, supple skin. Without adequate amounts of essential fatty acids, dry skin and conditions resembling eczema and psoriasis can occur.

Finally, copper depletes vitamin C, which together with the bioflavonoids is essential for collagen formation, capillary strength, and healing. Because of this vitamin C link, severe bruising often occurs in individuals with copper overload. Aestheticians I talk to at the International Cosmetology Conferences I speak at tell me they see a lot of diffuse redness and skin sensitivity these days. I suspect these conditions may be due in large part to the growing prevalence of copper overload.

YEAST OVERGROWTH

Yeast overgrowth, whether systemic or localized in the vagina, can be caused by a variety of factors, but the most overlooked factor by far is copper overload. What's the connection?

Ironically, many copper-toxic women find themselves troubled by a simultaneous excess and shortage of copper. They have high levels of copper stored in their tissues, but the copper is in an unbound form and therefore biounavailable—that is, the body isn't able to access the copper and properly use it. This phenomenon contributes to yeast overgrowth, because copper is the body's natural yeast killer. If copper is in a form that can't be readily used, the blood becomes deficient in copper and the white blood cells find their ability to kill off yeast diminished, setting the stage for yeast infections to develop.

While copper is necessary for yeast control, an excess of bioavailable copper can also cause problems: it's been shown to increase the pathogenic nature of the most common yeast organism, *Candida albicans*. Too much copper can therefore cause yeast infections to spread and worsen in intensity.

Optimal copper levels in blood and tissues are essential for both preventing and controlling the overgrowth of yeast. Many of my clients who had persistent yeast infections that didn't respond well to medical treatment found that their yeast problems disappeared after they went through my program to overcome copper overload.

PREMENSTRUAL SYNDROME

Researchers have long suspected that too much estrogen and not enough progesterone underlie the condition of premenstrual syndrome (PMS). Tissue mineral analysis studies reveal that the majority of women who experience PMS show an elevated tissue copper level and/or markedly low zinc-to-copper-ratio. This makes sense, considering the fact that estrogen levels are closely linked to copper levels in the body; when the level of one rises, the other rises too. Progesterone, on the other hand, is closely associated with zinc. The symptoms of PMS are strikingly similar to those of copper overload: fatigue, depression, frontal headaches, emotional volatility, and food cravings.

One recent study found that women troubled by PMS have significantly low levels of zinc in the blood compared to women who don't have PMS. According to the author of that study, zinc deficiency might lead to a decrease in secretions of progesterone and natural endorphins. Endorphins are feel-good, opiate-like substances produced by neurons in the brain that modulate perception of pain, mood, and various cravings. Another study suggested that an afternoon drop in progesterone levels (presumably from eating a low-zinc lunch) might contribute especially to cravings for sweet and salty foods, which can lead to food binges. All this research supports what I've seen with my clients: when women who have PMS lower high tissue copper levels by boosting their zinc reserves, their estrogen and progesterone levels normalize and their PMS symptoms dramatically lessen or disappear. Leonid Wilson, M.D., and other practitioners who treat copper overload also have successfully treated many PMS patients this way.

IMMUNE SYSTEM DISORDERS

Copper has antifungal and antibacterial effects, while zinc has antiviral effects. The immune system requires a good balance of both zinc and copper to keep a person healthy and free of illness. Individuals who are plagued by chronic bacterial infections tend to have copper that's low or biounavailable, while those who have chronic viral infections typically have low zinc and high copper levels.

David L. Watts, D.C., Ph.D., of Trace Elements Laboratories in Addison, Texas, explains the strong connection between copper overload and viral infections in his book *Trace Elements and Other Essential Nutrients* (Trace Elements, 1995, p. 86):

Excessive tissue copper levels are often seen in people who have had a severe viral condition such as hepatitis and mononucleosis. Following these infections, copper levels may remain elevated for years. The symptoms of fatigue, lethargy, and depression often linger as well.

High tissue copper predisposes an individual to recurring viral infections. This pattern is frequently seen in individuals who have been diagnosed with Epstein-Barr, and/or cytomegalovirus. These viruses are known to be related to the Chronic Fatigue Syndrome (CFS). Often individuals with CFS will have great difficulty overcoming their condition unless they have their tissue copper levels evaluated and take appropriate measures to lower excessive levels.

Chronic fatigue syndrome is connected to copper overload in another way. Numerous studies have suggested a strong link between CFS and adrenal gland dysfunction; some practitioners believe that all individuals who have CFS have weak adrenal function. You might remember from the last chapter that adrenal burnout is a common consequence of copper overload. It's no coincidence that adrenal burnout and CFS are both characterized by a feeling of total exhaustion.

The story that follows is that of health journalist Melissa Diane Smith. She struggled for years with chronic fatigue syndrome before finding, after a long search, that overcoming copper overload was key to her recovery. Before I tell you how she recovered, though, let me tell you how copper overload and zinc deficiency insidiously developed, leading to a devastating condition.

Melissa's Story

Melissa had a few minor copper-related symptoms during stressful times in high school, but her real problems started when she left home and went off to college. "I had high standards and was totally engrossed in my journalism studies. I burned the midnight oil often to meet story deadlines," she recalls. "Out on my own for the first time, I also began to eat more quick processed foods on the run and also to drink alcohol. All of these factors, I now know, depleted zinc levels in my body."

A few years into college, Melissa entered what she calls a "tumultuous and stressful relationship," and shortly later, she came down with mononucleosis, the acute illness caused by the Epstein-Barr virus. Even after she recovered from mononucleosis, she found herself feeling more tired and anxious than she'd been before her illness.

After college, Melissa began working as a public relations writer for a health resort. Because of that connection, she started eating a spa-type diet high in zinc-depleting carbohydrates and low in zinc-rich meats. "That diet was totally wrong for me," she says. Then, in the span of a few months, she was exposed to an excessive amount of stress at work and a flurry of chemicals—everything from pesticides sprayed in her home to components of the new carpet installed in her office. These stressors apparently were the final straws that caused her immune system to falter. Over the Labor Day weekend of 1987, Melissa developed what felt like a very bad flu, complete with severe sore throat, achy joints and muscles, chills, and utter exhaustion. "I thought it would go away after several days or a week," Melissa recounts, "but weeks passed, then months passed, and I still felt the same way." Her fatigue became so severe that she stopped working and tried to sleep and rest more, as her doctors had advised, but even that didn't seem to help much.

For the next two and a half years, Melissa saw nine doctors, all of whom either did nothing for her or gave her drugs that made her feel worse. "The sixth doctor I saw insinuated that I was a little 'psychologically off' because he couldn't find anything wrong with me. This infuriated me, because I knew deep in my heart that there was a real reason behind my health problems," she recalls. "Of *course* I was depressed, but the depression I had was mainly because I was so exhausted that I couldn't work, exercise, socialize, or have any kind of normal life."

Frustrated beyond belief, Melissa turned to the investigative research skills she'd learned in college to get to the bottom of her health problems. She delved into the study of nutrition and experimented with many "light" diets, but the lighter the diet she ate, the sicker and more tired she became. "I figured there must be a reason why the 'light' diet made me feel so bad—something health professionals hadn't clued in on."

Eventually she was diagnosed with chronic Epstein-Barr virus and learned that zinc deficiency was part of her problem. Then she uncovered bits and pieces of information about copper overload and, learning that she fit the copper overload profile perfectly, had a tissue mineral analysis performed. On her first several tests, high copper levels didn't show up because the copper was stored so deep in her tissues. (Melissa had what we call "hidden" copper overload. This condition usually occurs when the metabolism is very slow and when copper has been slowly building for a long time. You'll learn more about hidden copper overload in the next chapter.)

"Even though the copper levels weren't high on my tissue analysis, my zinc levels were low, and my intuition told me quite strongly that copper overload was the source of my health problems," Melissa says. She trusted her intuition and started a copper-control diet and built up her zinc reserves. Over the course of several years, her body gradually eliminated the copper that had built up in her tissues, and her fatigue and viral symptoms slowly but surely lifted.

"The recovery process wasn't easy—I had several difficult times when I experienced distressful symptoms because of 'copper dumps' [something you'll read about in Chapter 10]," Melissa explains. "But the copper-control program truly was a lifesaver for me. I feel quite certain that I wouldn't have recovered from chronic fatigue syndrome any other way."

Melissa had a severe case of copper overload; I had a relatively mild one. Melissa experienced viral symptoms, exhaustion, and depression; I experienced a tired body, mental racing, anxiety, insomnia, and skin problems. What our two stories show is that copper overload can manifest itself in countless ways, depending on the individual. Fatigue is always a factor in copper overload, but numerous other combinations of symptoms typically are involved.

In the next section, Part II, you'll learn how to test for copper overload and discover how to reverse the condition with diet, supplements, and stress management.

Part II

Treating Your Fatigue at the Source: Reversing Copper Overload

Chapter Seven

Testing for the Copper Connection to Your Fatigue

Determining whether copper overload is the culprit behind your fatigue can be tricky. As mentioned in Chapter 2, most health practitioners are taught to believe that copper overload takes only two forms: acute copper poisoning and Wilson's disease. When symptoms point to acute copper toxicity, traditional physicians perform tests that can detect these extreme cases, but those tests aren't helpful for detecting the subclinical tissue copper overload that causes so many cases of fatigue today. This testing failure explains why most people who suffer from copper overload don't know it, and why so many of us walk around feeling tired and lousy but can't say why. It's important to understand that just because *standard* medical tests don't show copper excess, you can't necessarily assume that you don't have copper overload. (Keep in mind that a frequent criticism of conventional medicine is its inability to detect subtle forms of chronic illness. Many women, for example, have all the clinical signs of hypothyroidism—that is, low thyroid function—but most of these women test negative for hypothyroidism on standard thyroid-function blood tests. Other, more sensitive thyroid-function tests used in alternative medicine often reveal that these women do in fact have the low thyroid function they suspected.)

The truth is that diagnosing copper overload, as with diagnosing most conditions, is more of an art than a science. Several different copper-assessing medical tests exist, but each has drawbacks and needs to be analyzed and interpreted correctly by a practitioner who has experience working with the condition of copper imbalance. To help you and your health practitioner diagnose copper overload, I offer here a quick rundown of what you need to know about the most common diagnostic tests that measure copper.

BLOOD TESTS

A serum (or blood) copper test, as you might gather, measures the amount of copper in the blood at the moment the blood sample was drawn. This test can be useful in some cases. Consistently low levels of serum copper or decreased levels of ceruloplasmin (a copper binding protein in the blood), for example, can be common indicators of Wilson's disease. High levels of copper in the blood, on the other hand, can indicate acute copper poisoning, but they can mean other things as well.

If copper overload is suspected, most physicians will only perform a blood test, but there are several problems with this method of detection. First, in my experience, most people who have high *tissue* copper levels have normal copper levels in the *blood*. This isn't surprising, because the body works hard to keep the levels of nutrients in the bloodstream within fairly tight limits. If large fluctuations in mineral levels occurred, serious illness or even death would result. So if we're exposed to a one-time episode of serious environmental copper—from copper-contaminated water, for example—levels of copper in the blood will rise to a certain point and then stop; any excess that can't be excreted is then stored away in tissues to prevent toxic amounts in the blood.

Another drawback to a blood test is that mineral levels in blood can vary slightly depending on the time of day, meals that we've eaten, our activity level, and other factors. A serum copper test measures the amount of copper in the blood in a brief moment in time, so it gives a short-term view of what's happening in the body, but not the long-term picture.

URINALYSIS

Some physicians use urinalysis as a tool in detecting extreme copper overload. Like blood tests, urinalysis generally isn't helpful for detecting most types of copper overload, however. Its usefulness is restricted to diagnosing or ruling out the extreme case of Wilson's disease (which is usually characterized by low levels of ceruloplasmin and high levels of copper in urine samples). If someone in your family has Wilson's disease—or if you have unexplained brain, neurological, or psychiatric dysfunctions, liver abnormalities, or gold or greenish-gold rings in your corneas—it's important for you to see your doctor to be tested for Wilson's disease.

TISSUE MINERAL ANALYSIS

Tissue mineral analysis is a simple, noninvasive screening test that reveals something very different than a blood test, ceruloplasmin test, or urinalysis. It provides a unique reading of the mineral levels in the cells over a two- to three-month period. Just as rings of a tree can reveal a tremendous amount of information about the climate and the condition of the soil a tree grew in years before it was cut, a hair sample—hair is the tissue of choice for this test—provides a long-term blueprint of what has occurred, metabolically speaking, in the cells. This is important, because it's in the cells—not in the blood or the urine—that energy is produced and that most metabolic activity takes place. Mineral levels in hair samples taken for tissue mineral analysis are about ten times the mineral levels in blood, so the detection of many conditions, including copper overload, is easier and more accurate with the hair-sample method. (To get an idea of how helpful this test can be, think about this: researchers using tissue mineral analysis determined, more than 100 years after his death, that Napoleon Bonaparte had been poisoned with arsenic. Although his hair was tested more than a century after his death, it still revealed pathological amounts of the arsenic that had gradually proved fatal.)

I'm fully aware that a lot of controversy surrounds the use of tissue mineral analysis; in fact, many practitioners dismiss it outright. But my experience over the past ten years has convinced me that it has unparalleled value in subclinical assessment of mineral levels. I've found it to be one of the best methods available for detecting both direct and hidden copper imbalance. To clear up some of the confusion surrounding tissue analysis, consider these important points raised by Larry Wilson, M.D., in *Nutritional Balancing and Hair Mineral Analysis: A Comprehensive Guide* (Wilson Consultants, 1991):

- Hair analysis laboratories are scrutinized more closely by the government than most blood laboratories. The U.S. Department of Health and Human Services, Health Care Financing Administration, Division of Health Standards and Quality carefully inspects each commercial hair analysis laboratory annually, and an operating license is issued only if personnel and procedures meet rigorous standards.
- Some laboratories wash hair before testing mineral levels and others don't. This difference in the handling of the hair can produce variable results. Washing the hair at the laboratory removes some of the loosely bound minerals and can reduce some mineral readings by 50 percent or more. To ensure the most accurate mineral readings, be sure your practitioner sends your hair sample to a federally licensed laboratory that does *not* wash the hair at the lab.
- Beauty parlor permanent-wave and hair-coloring treatments can affect hair mineral readings, because they alter hair structure. After having one of these treatments done, it's best to let the hair grow out for a few months (if possible) before having a hair sample taken. (The sample is always a snippet of the most recently grown inch to inch and a half of hair, taken from the back of the head.)
- Routine use of shampoos, conditioners, and rinses, as well as light perspiration and air pollution, don't significantly affect hair mineral readings. Daily swimming in pools, though, can cause artificially high copper readings.

A copper level exceeding 2.5 milligrams per one hundred grams of hair (or 2.5 mg %) is considered elevated. In the absence of external contamination (such as would result from daily swimming in pools or daily work in a copper mine), elevated hair copper has been proven to be a clinically meaningful screening test for copper toxicity.

The main drawback of tissue mineral analysis is that most practitioners aren't trained in how to correctly interpret test results. They take the test at face value and miss cases of "hidden" copper overload—cases that can be recognized only by someone trained in tissue analysis interpretation.

HIDDEN COPPER OVERLOAD

It may seem surprising, but many people who have copper overload don't initially test high in copper on tissue analysis. Their metabolisms are so depressed that the copper is tightly stored in tissues; it hasn't yet been released into circulation and deposited in the hair. Yet if they begin treatment for copper overload, eating a low-copper, high-zinc diet and taking supplements to boost the metabolism, copper will be mobilized from storage depots and show up in high amounts on tissue analysis conducted after several months. Because of copper's tendency to lurk undetected in tissues, practitioners need to look at other readings that can signal copper overload before it presents itself.

Probably the best way to evaluate true copper status is by looking not only at an individual's copper level but also at his or her zinc-to-copper ratio. If that ratio is very low—even if the copper level is low or normal—excess copper is likely to be lurking in the tissues. Several other readings on a tissue mineral test often indicate hidden copper toxicity, as you can see below:

Signs of Hidden Copper Overload in Tissue Mineral Analysis

Zinc-to-copper ratio of less than 6:1
Calcium higher than 100 mg %
Copper lower than 1 mg %
Potassium lower than 3 mg %
Mercury greater than 0.4 mg %
Sodium-to-potassium ratio of less than 2.2:1
Calcium-to-potassium ratio of greater than 10:1

Source: Larry Wilson, M.D., Nutritional Balancing and Hair Mineral Analysis

The more of these indicators that are found on a tissue analysis, the greater the likelihood there is of hidden copper overload.

As with most other tests, a tissue mineral analysis is helpful only if the results are evaluated correctly. To help your health practitioner learn the finer details of detecting copper overload through tissue mineral analysis, suggest that he or she contact one of the laboratories or nutrition training organizations named in the Resources section of this book. Appendix A also is a resource for you and your physician: it shows four examples of tissue mineral analysis that indicate either high copper levels or signs of hidden copper overload.

If you're interested in getting a tissue mineral analysis conducted on a hair sample but have trouble finding a doctor who will perform this service, call Uni Key Health Systems at 800-888-4353. Uni Key does not do tissue mineral analysis directly but can help connect you with a lab that does.

THE IMPORTANCE OF ASSESSING SYMPTOMS AND INDICATORS

Tests can be helpful in many cases, but how a person feels is the most important indicator to me of whether copper overload is involved. I've found that medical tests simply aren't as sophisticated as the wisdom of our bodies. If a client's symptoms and risk factors seem to indicate copper overload, I typically advise the client to follow the Energy-Revitalizing Diet outlined in the next two chapters and to take a copper-free multiple for a trial period of time. More often than not, these clients come back to me and say that they feel dramatically better. Their bodies have told them in no uncertain terms that the copper-control program was exactly what they needed to bring them back into balance and restore their energy.

Because of my belief in the importance of each client's perception of his or her health, I designed the copper overload questionnaire that follows. Taking this questionnaire will help you do with yourself what I do with clients in my practice—assess common symptoms and indicators associated with copper overload. If you answer yes to three or more questions in the quiz, some degree of copper overload is likely contributing to your fatigue and poor health.

Copper Overload Questionnaire

To get a good indication of whether you have copper overload, take the following quiz.

1. Do you eat frequent light meals but still lack energy?
   yes _____ *no* _____

2. Does your mind tend to race, even when your body is exhausted? *yes* _____ *no* _____

3. Do you consider yourself a highly creative person, but one who is frequently anxious and drained of energy? *yes* _____ *no* _____

4. Do you tend to daydream and live in your head?
   yes _____ *no* _____

5. Do you frequently experience insomnia because your mind simply won't calm down? *yes* _____ *no* _____

6. Are you prone to emotional and physical highs and lows?
   yes _____ *no* _____

7. Do you have frequent colds and flus, slow wound healing, lack of taste or appetite, or white spots on your fingernails?
   yes _____ *no* _____

8. Do you suffer from any of the following conditions—migraine headaches, hyperactivity, panic attacks, mood swings, depression, premenstrual tension, or skin problems—for which no underlying cause has been identified? *yes* _____ *no* _____

9. Do you have high estrogen levels or use the birth control pill, estrogen replacement therapy, or a copper IUD?
   yes _____ *no* _____

10. Do you either crave or adversely react to high-copper foods such as chocolate, nuts, avocados, and soy products?
    yes _____ *no* _____

11. Does your hair have a natural orange-red tint or copper-colored highlights? *yes* _____ *no* _____

12. Do you have dark areas of pigmentation or skin blotches on your face? *yes* _____ *no* _____

If you have three to five affirmative answers, you probably have some degree of copper overload.

If you have six to eight affirmative answers, it's very likely you have copper overload.

If you have nine to twelve affirmative answers, you almost certainly suffer a strong or long-standing case of copper overload.

UNDERSTANDING THE INDICATORS

1. If you feel that you're eating a healthy diet but are still tired, assume that you're not following the right advice for *you*. No one health regimen works for everyone. In my experience, the main group of people for whom frequent, light, mostly plant-based meals are *not* right are women who have copper overload. Meals consisting of legumes, whole grains, nuts, and especially soy products are healthy for some people, but not for those with copper overload. Because these foods are high in copper, they can cause or exacerbate copper buildup, thereby diminishing energy.

2. The combination of overactive mind and tired body is a tell-tale sign of copper overload. Here's why: copper is a brain stimulant. It speeds up mental processing, so high levels usually lead to racing thoughts. But high levels also stress the thyroid and adrenals, which are the glands most responsible for giving us get-up-and-go. When their functioning falters, energy is zapped. The result is a person who has all sorts of ideas racing through his or her mind but is too chronically exhausted to act on them.

3. Tissue mineral experts have noted that individuals who have high tissue copper levels tend to be right-brain dominant; in other words, they're intuitive, emotionally oriented, and artistically inclined. These individuals often have careers that involve creativity—careers in art, theater, music, and writing, for example. There are many advantages to being right-brain dominant as long as copper levels are kept

in check, but if copper levels rise too high, right-brainers often feel overemotional and anxious.

4. As mentioned earlier, copper excess can lead to mental over-activity. Indeed, people with copper overload sometimes are so wrapped up in their thoughts and daydreams that they're considered "spacey." According to some health profession-als who've worked with copper overload, high copper levels may serve as a defense mechanism that helps a sensitive individual cope with stress by allowing him or her to detach slightly from reality. This characteristic can inspire artistic creation and work well—as long as the copper doesn't rise too high.

5. Insomnia—especially hard-to-treat insomnia—is often an indicator of copper overload. As we saw earlier, copper is a brain stimulant, so excess copper typically interferes with sleep: people with copper overload often have trouble both falling asleep (because the mind won't relax) and staying asleep (because stimulating thoughts plague them in the middle of the night). These sleep problems can be particu-larly pronounced when a person is under a lot of stress, which causes copper levels to rise in the body and zinc levels to fall, thus exacerbating the tendency of a person with cop-per overload to have difficulty getting a good night's sleep.

6. Copper stimulates both mental and emotional overactivity, so those of us with high copper tend to be bright and cre-ative but also prone to emotional highs and lows. Often people with copper overload are so stimulated by their cre-ative ideas that they become emotionally and physically hyperactive for a while, drawing on borrowed energy despite their fundamental fatigue. When that fatigue catches up with them, they tend to come crashing down to a low in which they feel physically and emotionally wiped out.

7. Frequent colds and flus, slow wound healing, lack of taste or appetite, and white spots on fingernails are all typical

signs of zinc deficiency, a common factor that leads to the development of copper overload. As mentioned earlier, zinc is copper's primary antagonist, so without adequate zinc in the body, copper tends to build up simply because there's nothing to stop it. If you have any of these common zinc-deficiency symptoms, the chances are good that you have copper overload (or at least a copper-zinc imbalance).

8. Migraine headaches, hyperactivity, panic attacks, mood swings, depression, premenstrual tension, and skin problems are all symptoms frequently experienced by women, and each of these conditions has been associated with high levels of copper in the body. If you have any of these symptoms and haven't been able to find a cause for or relief from them, it's very likely that copper overload is involved.

9. High estrogen levels or use of the birth control pill, estrogen replacement therapy, or a copper IUD are strong risk factors for developing copper overload. Estrogen and copper levels tend to go hand in hand in the body; as the level of one rises, the level of the other tends to rise too. Researchers don't know exactly why there's such a close relationship between the two, but the current thinking is as follows: high copper levels diminish liver function, and a healthy liver is needed to break down estrogen each month to prevent estrogen buildup; high estrogen levels also diminish liver function, and a healthy liver is needed to excrete excess copper and prevent copper buildup. If you're on the pill or estrogen replacement therapy, or if you use a copper IUD, I urge you to have your copper levels checked regularly with tissue mineral analysis and avoid excessive copper in your diet.

10. Individuals with copper overload tend to either crave foods high in copper or have adverse reactions to them. Although it's a bit difficult to understand, many people who have high copper in their *tissues* have difficulty utilizing that stored copper. As a result, they become somewhat deficient in copper in their blood. Because of that deficiency, they

often crave high-copper foods to give them a temporary energy high. The new copper they ingest can't be utilized properly either, however, so instead of being circulated in the bloodstream, it's simply stored away, contributing further to the overload problem. This scenario is especially common among women right before their period. They often crave something like chocolate because they get a temporary emotional and physical lift from it, but then a while later they feel worse, experiencing a headache, lethargy, anxiety, or depression—conditions brought on by the additional copper.

11. Tissue mineral experts have noticed that people who have high copper levels often have red hair or a natural red or copper tint to blond or brown hair. (I know this sounds odd, but professionals who work with copper overload have definitely found it to be the case!) The exact details of how copper affects hair color are not known, but we do know that copper has a role in the formation of melanin, a pigmentary substance that influences the color of hair. Many of my clients report that when they look back to the onset of their copper overload symptoms, they remember that their hair color developed an uncharacteristically orange-red or copper tint.

12. Just as copper-dependent melanin influences the color of hair, so too does it influence the color of skin. Dark areas of pigmentation or skin blotches on the face often are signs of hidden copper overload. This unusual pigmentation is most likely to occur during pregnancy, when estrogen and copper levels rise. During this time, some women develop what doctors call a "pregnancy mask"—dark areas on the face, especially above the lip and on the lower forehead. The dark pigmentation also can be seen occasionally in nonpregnant women who have high estrogen and copper levels.

It's important to understand that copper buildup is much more common in women than men: the higher estrogen levels women have increase the likelihood of copper buildup. Women also usually have slower metabolisms than men, and the slower the metabolism of an individual, the less efficient the body is at eliminating excess copper. So women are much more likely to experience copper overload. Statistics from Trace Elements, Inc., a tissue mineral analysis lab in Addison, Texas, show that females between 30 and 48 years of age who send their hair in for analysis have high copper levels or low zinc-to-copper ratios about five times more often than males of the same age.

TRUSTING YOUR INTUITION

Having been introduced to the common indicators of copper over-load, you probably now have a good idea of whether that condition is a factor behind the fatigue you're experiencing. There's one other good "test" you can take to see whether a copper-focused energy-revitalizing program might be right for you. Think back to what you read in earlier chapters of this book. Do certain stories or symptoms ring true for you? Most of my clients, after learning about this syndrome, seem to get a strong sense of whether hidden copper overload is the missing link to the problems they've been experiencing. If you get this sense, your intuition is probably right! Read on to find out how to design a diet that will give you the energy advantage you've been searching for.

Chapter Eight

Basics of the Energy-Revitalizing Diet

The Energy-Revitalizing Diet is uniquely designed to rebuild energy by helping the body overcome copper overload. The diet combines complex carbohydrates, protein, and fat at each meal to keep blood sugar balanced throughout the day. This encourages a consistent, steady energy level and strengthens adrenal function, which is vital for recovering from copper overload. It also includes a strategy you haven't seen in other diets: an emphasis on zinc-rich foods and an avoidance of both high-copper foods and zinc-depleting foods. This three-step strategy helps bring copper back into the proper balance with zinc; and when zinc and copper levels are balanced, energy returns.

Most of us have never thought about foods in terms of their copper and zinc content, so this perspective usually requires some retraining. Instead of thinking about the calorie or fat content of various foods, as many Americans now do, you need to shift your focus to how different foods affect copper and zinc status. What follows is a rundown of the basic guidelines you need to understand as you shift your focus. (For a detailed listing of the amounts of copper and zinc in many common foods, see Appendix E.)

PROTEIN

Adequate dietary protein is critical for both preventing and overcoming copper overload. Protein helps boost metabolism by stimulating thyroid and adrenal function, it enhances the detoxification of excess copper and other toxins by the liver, and it's the central component of protein carriers, which allow for the proper transport and utilization of copper.

Protein also plays a crucial role in maintaining steady blood sugar and energy levels. It stimulates production of glucagon, a hormone that (taking the opposite role to insulin) promotes the burning of fat for energy. It also assists the body in absorbing and retaining zinc, a nutrient that's vital not only for blood sugar balance but also for preventing and reversing copper overload. Protein is important for so many reasons that it's best to eat small amounts throughout the day—preferably at every single meal and snack. If you have trouble eating this much protein, start with whatever amount you can tolerate and gradually add more protein to your diet as you're able to.

Land-Based Animal Protein (Eggs, Poultry, and Meats)

Land-based animal protein sources—eggs, poultry, wild game, and red meats—are our best sources of zinc. It's vital to include these protein sources in the diet to help reverse copper overload or to correct zinc deficiency or copper-zinc imbalance.

These days many people avoid red meats because of concerns about fat. People with copper overload do have trouble digesting fat, but they also desperately need rich dietary sources of zinc and protein. To assist the body in overcoming copper overload, the best game plan is to emphasize low-fat sources of zinc-rich animal protein, especially eggs, chicken, turkey, and game meats such as venison when available. Also try to include dark-meat poultry and lean cuts of red meats—such as ground round, sirloin steak, and flank steak—a few times a week, if you can tolerate them. Although dark-meat poultry and red meats contain more fat than white-meat poultry and can be harder to digest, they also contain significantly more zinc.

If you have trouble digesting meats—red meats in particular—try taking hydrochloric acid capsules or plant-based digestive enzymes with meals to assist the digestion process. These enzyme products often help prevent or lessen the "heavy" feeling that's common in the digestive tract after individuals with copper overload eat animal protein.

There are three caveats to keep in mind regarding land-based animal protein. The first is to try to buy organic meats and eggs whenever possible. The zinc in meats and eggs is essential for recovering from copper overload, but the antibiotics and hormones fed to commercial animals can indirectly contribute to copper buildup.

Protein is critical for recovery from copper overload, but it's possible to overeat protein. The body can absorb only so much protein in one sitting, so keep portion sizes moderate—about the size of your palm or a deck of cards. It's best to spread small amounts of protein throughout the day—at two different meals at least. It's also important to balance meats with fiber-rich vegetables to prevent constipation.

Finally, stick with muscle meats rather than organ meats. Although organ meats (such as liver and brain) are rich in many nutrients, they're harmful to those with copper overload because they're incredibly high in copper. (Just as copper can accumulate in our liver and brain, so too can it accumulate in the liver and brain of animals.)

Water-Based Animal Protein (Fish and Shellfish)

Fish is a good source of lean protein that's low in copper and easy to digest. These attributes make it a good protein choice for many copper-toxic individuals, especially former vegetarians, who need protein to enhance detoxification but have trouble digesting other forms of animal protein. Fish is not particularly rich in zinc, however, so it's not as beneficial for correcting zinc deficiency or copper-zinc imbalance as meat is. To assist the body in eliminating excess copper, emphasize zinc-rich, land-based animal protein in your diet, but include easy to digest fish at least several times a week.

Shellfish such as shrimp, lobster, and crab are good for many people because they're low in fat and rich in many nutrients, including zinc. Unfortunately, shellfish aren't good for those of us who are copper-toxic; the high copper content of shellfish can be problematic for those who have trouble eliminating excess copper. Individuals with copper overload should avoid all shellfish, but especially oysters, which contain 17 milligrams of copper per three-and-a-half-ounce serving—an amount that can be outright dangerous for copper-toxic individuals.

Dairy Products

Dairy products don't contain a lot of either zinc or copper, but they should be minimized in the diet because they can indirectly contribute to copper overload in a variety of ways. First, they contain high amounts of calcium, a mineral that tends to slow down the metabolism. Many dairy foods—cheese and ice cream, for example—are high in fat, which further slows the metabolism. (The slower the metabolism of the individual, you might remember, the more prone the person is to copper accumulation.)

The large amounts of calcium in dairy products are particularly problematic when consumed in conjunction with large amounts of phytic acid, which is found in grains and soy foods. Phytic acid is a compound that inhibits zinc absorption, and the combination of high calcium intake and high phytic acid intake decreases zinc absorption even more. To prevent zinc deficiency or a slowdown of body metabolism that can sabotage the body's ability to overcome copper overload, select low-fat and nonfat dairy products and use them sparingly—as flavoring condiments rather than as centerpieces in meals and snacks. Especially avoid eating combinations of high-fat dairy foods such as cheese together with grains or soy foods—combinations such as macaroni and cheese, tofu lasagna, tofu/dairy desserts, and so on.

Plant Protein Sources (Soy Products, Nuts and Seeds, and Legumes)

As a group, plant sources of protein should be greatly reduced in the diet of those trying to reverse copper overload. This is because legumes (beans and peas), soy foods, and nuts and seeds all provide less of the essential amino acids we need than animal foods do; in other words, they provide a lower-quality protein. Too little protein in the diet can cause adrenal and liver function to become sluggish; and when adrenal and liver function diminish, copper detoxification declines. Vegetable protein sources also contain significant amounts of copper, and recent research shows that when copper intake in the diet is high, considerable copper is retained in the body.

Soy foods have unusually high amounts of copper, and they also contain phytic acid. This means that soy foods are double trouble for those trying to overcome copper overload or copper-zinc imbalance and should therefore be strictly avoided.

All nuts and seeds, with one exception, also are high in copper and should be avoided. The exception is pumpkin seeds. Pumpkin seeds do contain copper, but they're incredibly rich in zinc and have a good zinc-to-copper balance. If your overall diet is low in copper, pumpkin seeds can be eaten in small amounts several times a week to help boost zinc status. One delicious way to include more pumpkin seeds in your diet is by eating a product called Pumpkorn for a snack. The maple-vanilla variety of Pumpkorn is soy-free, and I highly recommend it for those with copper overload. (To find out where you can purchase Pumpkorn in your area or to order the product directly, call Mental Processes, Inc., at 800-431-4018.)

Legumes, another source of plant protein, also contain copper, though not in the quantities found in soy products, nuts, and seeds. They also supply sulfur-rich amino acids, which are needed to enhance liver detoxification. Thus legumes, like pumpkin seeds, can be a helpful addition to the diet when eaten occasionally and in small amounts.

CARBOHYDRATES

Carbohydrates perform many valuable functions and are important, in *moderation,* to promote recovery from copper overload. When carbohydrates are balanced with protein in the diet, absorption of zinc, copper's primary antagonist, improves, and metabolism is revved up. Both of these outcomes—improved absorption of zinc and faster metabolism—enhance the copper detoxification process. If the diet is high in carbohydrates and low in protein, however, zinc absorption and retention diminish and copper is more likely to build up.

Vegetables

The main type of carbohydrates that should be emphasized in the diet is vegetables. As a group, vegetables supply the lowest amount of carbohydrates per serving, and they release glucose slowly, contributing to steady blood sugar and energy levels (and thereby minimizing stress on the adrenal glands). They also are low in copper (with the exception of mushrooms) and rich in fiber, both of which encourage detoxification of excess copper. Vegetables don't supply much zinc, but they form the perfect counterpart to zinc-rich meats, because they don't interfere with zinc absorption and they help prevent the constipation that can occur from eating meat. To encourage copper elimination, balance your intake of animal protein at meals with a liberal consumption of vegetables—at least one to two cups of raw vegetables or one-half to one cup of cooked vegetables several times a day.

Although most vegetables can be eaten liberally, there are a few that should be limited in the diet. Starchy vegetables such as potatoes, carrots, and corn are converted to glucose quickly and therefore can cause quick blood sugar highs followed by quick blood sugar lows. Erratic blood sugar levels tax adrenal and liver function, and this in turn can interfere with the body's utilization and detoxification of copper. To promote steady blood sugar, eat starchy vegetables only occasionally. Limit yourself to the serving sizes listed below and make sure you balance the starchy vegetables you eat in meals and snacks with animal protein and small amounts of fat.

Serving Portions for Starchy Vegetables

Chestnuts, roasted	4 large or 6 small
Corn (cooked)	1/2 cup
Corn (on the cob)	1 (4 inches long)
Parsnips	1 small
Potatoes, white (baked or boiled)	1 small
Potatoes, white (mashed)	1/2 cup
Pumpkin	3/4 cup
Rutabaga	1 small
Squash (winter types)	1/2 cup
Succotash	1/2 cup

Legumes

Legumes, a source of carbohydrates as well as protein, trigger slow rises in blood sugar levels, helping to promote steady energy, but they're higher in carbohydrates and higher in copper than vegetables. Therefore, while legumes can be eaten occasionally, the amount eaten in one sitting should be controlled.

Serving Portions for Legumes

Beans: lima, navy, pinto, kidney, garbanzo, black (dried, cooked)	1/2 cup
Beans (baked, plain)	1/2 cup
Lentils (dried, cooked)	1/4 cup
Peas (dried, cooked)	1/2 cup
Peas (split)	1/4 cup

Grains

Grains—both the refined varieties and whole grains—adversely affect copper-zinc balance when they're eaten excessively. As you'll recall from Chapter 3, white flour is stripped of most of its zinc in the refining process; the same is true of white rice. Because zinc is needed to digest and metabolize carbohydrates, eating low-zinc refined-grain products can contribute to zinc deficiency—which of course increases the likelihood of copper buildup. Refined-grain products also have most of their fiber removed in the refining process, and lack of fiber in the diet can lead to irregularity and sluggish elimination of copper. To encourage copper detoxification and general good health, I recommend eliminating zinc- and fiber-deficient refined-grain products (that is, white-flour breads, muffins, bagels, croissants, pretzels, and so on) from the diet as much as possible.

Unrefined whole grains have their bran and germ intact, so they contain much more zinc than white-flour products; however, the zinc they contain isn't absorbed well because of the zinc-inhibiting phytic acid and insoluble fiber that are also present. Whole grains—whole wheat, in particular—have another knock against them: they contain significant amounts of copper, which can be problematic for those trying to reverse copper overload. To enhance copper elimination, be sure to avoid wheat bran and wheat germ, which are very high in copper, and do your best to avoid or minimize whole-wheat products (breads, tabouli, tortillas, baked goods). Many copper overload experts have noticed that copper-toxic individuals tend to be sensitive to whole-wheat products and sometimes to whole wheat's close relatives, spelt and kamut. When these grains are removed from the diet, the copper detoxification process seems to go more smoothly.

Grains other than whole-wheat products don't seem to be as problematic for individuals who have copper overload. However, like starchy vegetables, whole grains tend to cause blood sugar highs and lows, because they release glucose quickly into the bloodstream; and, like legumes, they contain significant amounts of copper. This means that whole grains and whole-grain products should be eaten infrequently; never eaten alone, but always balanced with zinc-rich protein and small amounts of fat; and monitored in terms of portion size.

Serving Portions for Grain Products

Cereals and Grains

Amaranth (cooked)	1/4 cup
Barley (cooked)	1/4 cup
Bran (unprocessed rice bran)	1/4 cup
Buckwheat groats (kasha, cooked)	1/4 cup
Cornmeal (cooked)	1/4 cup
Grits (cooked)	1/4 cup
Millet (cooked)	1/4 cup
Oat groats	1/4 cup
Oatmeal (steel-cut)	1/2 cup
Quinoa (cooked)	1/4 cup
Rice (brown, cooked)	1/4 cup
Rice (wild, cooked)	1/4 cup
Rye berries	1/4 cup
Rye, rolled	1/2 cup
Tapioca	2 Tbsp
Teff	1/2 cup

Flours

Arrowroot	2 Tbsp
Buckwheat	3 Tbsp
Cornmeal	2 Tbsp
Potato flour	2½ Tbsp
Rice flour	3 Tbsp

Pasta

Noodles (rice, cooked)	1/4 cup

Breads

Rye bread	1/2 slice
Tortilla, corn	1 (6 inches)

Crackers

Rice wafers (brown rice, Westbrae)	1 large
Ryvita Light or Dark Crisp Bread	1 to 1½ crackers
Wasa Light Rye Crisp Bread	2 crackers

Fruits

Fresh fruits are low in copper (and also in zinc); rich in fiber, which helps promote digestive regularity; and loaded with many antioxidants and phytochemicals that help protect health. As beneficial as fruits can be, however, they shouldn't be eaten with abandon. Fruits are simple sugars, so when they're eaten excessively, they can contribute to blood sugar problems, weak immunity, and yeast infections. Because individuals with copper overload and copper-zinc imbalance are prone to all three of these conditions, eating significant amounts of fruit can make it difficult to overcome copper-related health problems.

To accelerate recovery from copper overload, try to discipline yourself to eating only a serving or two of fruits a day, *after* well-balanced meals and snacks. If you suffer from severe blood sugar imbalance, weak immunity, or frequent viruses or yeast infections, cut down your intake of fruit even more. In severe cases, you may need to avoid fruit completely. Prunes, dates, raisins, and other dried fruits are concentrated sources of sugars and are quite high in copper. They particularly should be avoided.

Serving Portions for Fruits

Apple	1/2
Apple butter (sugar-free)	2 Tbsp
Apricots (fresh)	3
Banana	1/3
Berries: boysenberries, blackberries, blueberries, loganberries	1/2 cup
Cantaloupe	1/4 melon or 1 cup cubed
Cherries	7
Figs (fresh)	1 large
Fruit cocktail (canned in juice)	1/2 cup
Fruit preserves and spreads (sugar-free)	2 Tbsp
Grapefruit	1/2 small
Grapes	10
Honeydew melon, cubed	1/2 cup
Kiwi	1 medium
Lemon	1

Lime	1
Mango, sliced	1/3 cup
Nectarine	1/2
Orange	1/2
Papaya	1/2 cup
Peach	1 medium
Pear	1/3
Pineapple	1/2 cup
Plum	1
Raspberries	2/3 cup
Strawberries	3/4 cup
Tangerine	1 large
Watermelon	1/2 cup

Sugars and Sweets

Sugar is a definite no-no for those trying to overcome copper-related fatigue and other health problems. First, sugar actively depletes levels of zinc in the body. Second, it's absorbed extremely quickly into the bloodstream, causing blood sugar highs and lows that stress adrenal and pancreatic function and lead to further fatigue. This ultimate drop in energy usually results in intense cravings for sugar and refined carbohydrates for quick energy—and yet when we give in to our cravings and eat these foods, we further deplete zinc levels and diminish energy! Even more so than fruits, sugar and sugar-sweetened treats exacerbate blood sugar problems, weaken immunity, and contribute to yeast overgrowth. If you're serious about speeding up your recovery from copper overload and the unpleasant symptoms that come with it, strictly avoid both sugar-sweetened and naturally sweetened foods—including cookies, candy, muffins, fruit-juice-sweetened yogurt (and frozen yogurt), and pies and cakes. This may seem difficult, but if you're like many of my clients, you'll find it much easier to do when you eat a blood sugar–balancing diet rich in zinc and protein.

Once you begin the Energy-Revitalizing Diet, try to satisfy the occasional sweet tooth with fruit. If fruit doesn't seem to satisfy you, try a cookie or dessert that contains less than five grams of sugar per serving. Keep in mind that the worst dessert for those with copper overload is chocolate, which is extremely high in copper. If you're accustomed to eating a lot of sugar, avoiding sugar may be difficult at first, but continue to remind yourself that doing so will help the body recover more quickly from the conditions associated with copper overload or copper-zinc imbalance.

FATS

Often unfairly labeled the villains behind poor health, dietary fats play several important roles in recovery from copper overload. Fats are used by the body to make hormones, including the adrenal hormones, which help the body balance blood sugar and cope with stress, and those that stimulate proper utilization and detoxification of copper by the liver. Fats also slow down the entry of carbohydrates into the bloodstream, helping to promote long-term energy and greater satisfaction for long periods after meals. In addition, they increase eating enjoyment, because they carry compounds that give food much of its flavor and aroma. Eating small quantities of high-quality fats can therefore help individuals with copper overload stick to the Energy-Revitalizing Diet without feeling deprived and can assist the copper detoxification process by promoting blood sugar balance and healthy adrenal function.

Too much dietary fat, however, can lead to copper buildup. As discussed in an earlier chapter, individuals with copper overload typically have trouble metabolizing fats, because copper buildup interferes with liver function. By reversing copper overload, we can boost both fat digestion and fat metabolism. Individuals with copper overload usually have slow metabolisms generally, making the body less efficient at eliminating excess copper (regardless of copper intake). Since fat also tends to slow metabolism, eating an excessive amount of fat can interfere with copper detoxification and lead to more copper buildup. The solution to this problem is to eliminate unhealthy fats—the kinds many Americans unknowingly eat—replacing them with fats (used in small amounts) that promote health and are low in copper.

The *Really* Bad Fats

The fats that are real hazards to our health are called *trans fatty acids*. Found in margarine, vegetable shortening, deep-fried foods, and all convenience foods that list hydrogenated or partially hydrogenated oils on the label, these undesirable fats have been connected to heart disease, immune system suppression, reproductive problems, and a reduced ability of the body to rid itself of toxins and carcinogens. Most Americans, unaware of how harmful trans fatty acids are, eat these fats frequently in many processed foods. If you eliminate these fats from your diet, you'll promote better overall health and your fat intake will drop dramatically, usually leveling off to an amount that copper-toxic individuals do well on.

Vegetable Oils

Vegetable oils supply healthy fats for those trying to reverse copper overload, provided the right oils are used in the right ways. Most supermarket-quality oils are refined, which means they're heated at high temperatures, treated with solvents, bleached, and deodorized. These processing steps render refined vegetable oils almost as harmful to health as partially hydrogenated oils, and such refined products therefore should be avoided.

Vegetable oils that are labeled *unrefined,* on the other hand, are healthful. The techniques that are used to make unrefined vegetable oils protect delicate fatty acids in the oils from turning rancid or being damaged, and help keep the small amounts of fat-soluble vitamins found in the oils intact. As an added bonus, unrefined vegetable oils taste and smell like the nut, seed, or fruit from which they were derived, so they're much more flavorful than typical supermarket oils. Look for unrefined vegetable oils in health-food stores and natural-food supermarkets, and use them sparingly—no more than a teaspoonful at a time.

Some unrefined oils, such as sesame oil, are derived from nuts and seeds that are high in copper, but don't be concerned. When the oils are used in appropriately small amounts, the copper content is negligible and not problematic.

It's important to understand that the more unsaturated an unrefined oil is, the more sensitive it is to destruction from heat and light. Flaxseed oil, for example, is rich in highly unsaturated omega-3 fatty acids that are essential for health, but these fatty acids are extremely sensitive to heat and light. This means that flaxseed oil should never be heated; it should only be used raw—on top of salads and cooked cereals, for example. Olive oil, on the other hand, is rich in heat-stable monounsaturated fatty acids and therefore is an excellent oil for cooking. Cold-pressed, extra-virgin olive oil—another unrefined option—is one of the best "good" fats to include in your diet.

Butter
Believe it or not, butter has a place in the Energy-Revitalizing Diet. A mostly saturated fat, butter stands up even better to high-temperature cooking than olive oil. Use it in very small amounts as a flavorful addition to the diet.

Nuts and Seeds
Nuts and seeds are a great source of healthy fats, but unfortunately they're quite high in copper. Although nuts and seeds are good blood sugar–stabilizing foods, most individuals trying to reverse copper overload should strictly avoid them until their condition improves. The only exception to this rule concerns pumpkin seeds. As mentioned in the protein discussion above, pumpkin seeds contain copper, but they're a rich source of zinc and have a good copper-zinc balance. They also supply omega-6 and omega-3 fatty acids, both of which are essential for health. Individuals with copper overload should therefore try to include a tablespoon or two of pumpkin seeds in their diet several times a week.

Fatty Fish
Fatty fish—a category that includes salmon, halibut, trout, tuna, and sardines—is primarily a protein source, but I've included it in this section on fat because it supplies EPA and DHA—two omega-3 essential fatty acids that are hard to obtain any other way. Like lean fish, fatty fish doesn't provide much zinc compared to land-based animal protein, but because it provides health-promoting omega-3 fatty acids, fatty fish should be eaten at least a few times each week.

Avocados
Because avocados are good sources of healthy fats and vitamin E, I recommend them for most people—but not for those with copper overload. Avocados are high in fat and copper, so they tend to slow down metabolism and contribute to copper accumulation. It's best to

avoid avocados when you're trying to reverse high tissue copper levels. As with nuts and seeds, though, you can gradually add small amounts of this food back into your diet once your copper levels normalize.

SEASONINGS

Herbs, spices, and seasonings contain small amounts of copper and zinc, but most don't affect copper and zinc status significantly. However, brewer's yeast—a popular topper for popcorn with many health-food enthusiasts—contains surprisingly high amounts of copper. Even small amounts of brewer's yeast should be avoided.

Because curry and black pepper also contain significant amounts of copper, some individuals with copper overload feel better after eliminating these seasonings from their diet. Ginger and cinnamon, on the other hand, are high-zinc spices; you might try sprinkling these seasonings on various foods as a way to help boost zinc status ever so slightly.

COOKWARE

As was noted in Chapter 4, copper cookware can leach small amounts of copper into foods. Over time, this additional source of copper can lead to copper buildup. To help prevent or reverse copper overload, avoid using copper cookware. Instead, choose pots and pans made from stainless steel, ceramic, or glass.

FLAVORED BEVERAGES

Since beverages are liquids, we tend to think they don't affect our nutritional status, but they do. Tea and iced tea, for example, are quite high in copper; so is beer. Coffee and high-sugar soft drinks act as zinc-zappers, while alcohol causes zinc to be flushed out of the system. Fruit juices are concentrated sources of sugar without the blood sugar–balancing fiber found in fruit, so they tend to cause blood sugar highs and lows that can stress adrenal, pancreatic, and liver function; compounding the problem, the fatigue caused by the stress of that blood sugar fluctuation increases the yen for sweets. Avoid all these drinks as much as possible to increase zinc status and promote optimal elimination of excess copper. The best drink to encourage detoxification is the only drink that's a nutrient unto itself—water. There's one catch, though: the water we drink needs to be low in copper and free of other common toxins.

WATER

Water, as we learned in Chapter 4, can contain high amounts of copper for a variety of reasons: because high amounts of copper occur naturally in the water supply; because copper compounds are added to the water supply to prevent fungi and algae growth; or because copper has leached from copper pipes into the water. A good indicator of high copper levels in the water from your tap is a blue-green ring on kitchen and bathroom fixtures. This isn't a foolproof sign, though; copper levels can be high even without that staining.

The only way to know for sure whether your water is contributing to bodily copper buildup and sabotaging your energy level is to test your water. For information on how to do this with an easy-to-use home water-testing kit, see Appendix B.

Taking the time to test your water and invest in a filter that reduces copper may be a hassle you'd rather avoid. But it's important to remember that we not only drink water and bathe in it, but we also cook our foods in it. Even if we strictly adhere to the Energy-Revitalizing Diet, if the water we use is high in copper, this alone may prevent us from overcoming copper-induced fatigue.

Chapter Nine

Following the
Energy-Revitalizing Diet

The previous chapter introduced the concepts underlying the Energy-Revitalizing Diet and offered general guidelines for reducing copper overload through nutrition. This chapter puts a more nuts-and-bolts spin on those guidelines, helping you to see—through sample menus and copper-reduced recipes—how the Energy-Revitalizing Diet can become part of your life.

Let's begin by reviewing foods that should be avoided or emphasized by people concerned about copper overload:

BRIEF LIST OF FOODS
TO AVOID AND EMPHASIZE

High-Copper Foods to Avoid

Soy products (soy-based protein powders, tofu, tempeh, soy sauce or tamari, most imitation meat products, soy milk, etc.)

Wheat bran and wheat germ

Yeast

Nuts, nut butters, and seeds (exception: pumpkin seeds)

Chocolate

Dried fruits

Mushrooms

Shellfish (lobster, shrimp, crab, scallops, etc.)
Organ meats such as liver
Tea

Zinc-Depletors to Avoid
Alcohol
Coffee
Sugar
Carbohydrates in excess, especially whole grains

Zinc-Rich Foods to Emphasize
Eggs
Chicken
Turkey
Red meats
Wild game
Pumpkin seeds

Let's look now at how foods low in copper and high in zinc can be combined in ways that maintain consistent blood sugar levels and sustain energy.

ONE-WEEK SAMPLE MENU PLAN—DAY ONE

BREAKFAST
Eggs Florentine (2 eggs scrambled in olive oil with spinach and
   onions)

LUNCH
Greek salad with cucumber, tomatoes, Bermuda onions, 2 tsp crum-
   bled goat cheese, and 1 Tbsp pumpkin seeds
Dressing of lemon juice, olive oil, garlic, and herbs

DINNER
Broiled Turkey-Vegetable Kabobs*[1]
^{1}/$_4$ cup cooked wild rice and brown rice pilaf

[1]An asterisk indicates that the recipe is provided later in this chapter.

DAY TWO

BREAKFAST

1 hard-boiled egg sprinkled lightly with Real Salt
1 wheat-free brown-rice waffle topped with 1/3 cup thawed frozen
    blueberries

LUNCH

Taco salad with 1 oz grilled seasoned chicken strips, 1 oz black beans,
    1 oz low-fat mozzarella cheese, diced onions, and cilantro on a
    large bed of green leaf lettuce, topped with salsa
Jicama sticks squeezed with lime

DINNER

Broiled halibut brushed with tarragon, olive oil, and lemon
Double serving of steamed asparagus
$^1/_4$ cup quinoa pilaf cooked in vegetable broth

DAY THREE

BREAKFAST

$^1/_2$ grapefruit
4 small Turkey Sausage Patties*
1 slice whole-grain-rye sourdough toast with 1 tsp butter

LUNCH

Tuna salad with 3 oz canned, flaked tuna and minced green onion,
    celery, and cilantro, mixed with 1 tsp Spectrum canola mayon-
    naise, served on green lettuce leaves
4 small carrot and celery sticks

DINNER

Zesty Ginger-Cinnamon Chicken Breast*
$^1/_2$ cup butternut squash, baked

DAY FOUR

BREAKFAST
$^1/_2$ cup oatmeal with $^1/_2$ chopped apple, ground cinnamon, a few
    teaspoons pumpkin seeds, and a drizzle of unrefined flaxseed
    oil

LUNCH
Broiled organic turkey burger, buffalo burger, or hamburger sprin-
    kled with garlic powder, served on red lettuce leaves with red onion
    slices and sliced tomato
1 small baked potato topped with chives and 1 tsp butter

DINNER
$^1/_2$ Roast Cornish Hen and Vegetable Stuffing Herbs de Provence*
Steamed brussels sprouts

DAY FIVE

BREAKFAST
2 poached eggs on hash-browned potatoes

LUNCH
Shelton-brand chicken chili
$^1/_2$ cup pineapple

DINNER
3 oz sliced roast turkey breast, au jus
$^1/_2$ baked sweet potato with 1 tsp butter and a dash of cinnamon
French-cut green beans

DAY SIX

BREAKFAST
4 turkey breast slices or Turkey Sausage Patties*
Hot cream-of-brown-rice cereal topped with sliced fresh peach and
    sprinkled with cinnamon

LUNCH
Romaine and baby mixed green salad topped with 3 oz broiled
  chicken strips
Dressing of lemon juice and olive oil

DINNER
Poached or broiled salmon with lemon
Vegetable medley of broccoli, cauliflower, and carrots

DAY SEVEN

BRUNCH
Brunch scramble with cubed turkey, cooked brown rice, rubbed sage,
  onions, parsley, spinach, and chicken broth

SNACK
Maple-Vanilla Pumpkorn (seasoned pumpkin seed snack)

DINNER
2 small broiled lamb chops seasoned with garlic, oregano, and lemon
Steamed artichoke with lemon, olive oil, garlic, and fresh basil dip-
  ping sauce

ZINC-RICH RECIPES

The following recipes are easy, zinc-rich entrées developed specifically
for copper overload, courtesy of nutritionist Melissa Diane Smith.

Turkey Sausage Patties
1 pound lean, organic ground turkey
2–6 garlic cloves, crushed and pressed
$^1/_2$ tsp rubbed sage
$^1/_2$ tsp ground fennel
Unrefined natural sea salt to taste (optional)

Preheat oven to 350 degrees. Mix the above ingredients, shape
the mixture into round 2-inch-diameter sausage patties, and

place on a broiler pan or on a wire rack above a baking pan.
Bake until done and no pink remains in the center, about
20–25 minutes. Add sea salt to taste at the table if necessary.
Serves 3 to 4 people.

Roast Cornish Hen and Vegetable Stuffing Herbs de Provence
1 Cornish hen, cut in half
1¹/₂ tsp unrefined extra-virgin olive oil
1 onion, diced
1 carrot, diced
1 stalk celery, diced
3 cloves garlic, minced
1 tsp sage
¹/₄–¹/₂ tsp herbs de Provence
1¹/₂ tsp chicken broth or water

In a large bowl, toss the hen halves and diced vegetables with
the olive oil and herbs. Mix well so that everything is moist.
Pour the chicken broth or water in the bottom of a baking pan;
then place the vegetable mixture in two separate mounds in the
pan. Top each mound with the Cornish hen half, folding as
much of the vegetable mixture as possible under the meat. Bake
at 350 degrees for 1 hour. Serves 2.

Broiled Turkey-Vegetable Kabobs
1¹/₂ lbs organic turkey breast cutlets, cut into 3/4-inch kabob
    cubes
Juice of 2 limes
1 Tbsp extra-virgin olive oil
1 cup chicken, vegetable, or turkey broth
¹/₂ tsp coriander
1¹/₂ tsp oregano
6 garlic cloves, finely minced
1 large zucchini, sliced into 1/4-inch rounds
1 large onion, chopped into kabob skewer pieces

Combine the lime juice, olive oil, broth, garlic, and seasonings
to make the marinade. Add the turkey, zucchini, and onion to

the marinade and marinate for at least 15 minutes. Remove
turkey cubes, zucchini, and onion from the marinade and
arrange on skewers, reserving the marinade. Brush some of the
marinade over the kabobs and broil them for about 10 minutes. Turn kabobs over, brush with more marinade, and broil
for another 10 minutes. If turkey is still pink in the middle, flip
over one more time, brush with more marinade, and broil for
an additional 5–10 minutes. Serves 4.

Zesty Ginger-Cinnamon Chicken Breasts
4 large organic boneless, skinless chicken breast halves
$1/2$ cup chicken broth (Pacific Foods of Oregon organic brand
    preferred)
1 tsp unrefined olive or sesame oil
2 tsp additional oil for browning
2 Tbsp fresh ginger root, peeled and finely chopped
3 garlic cloves, pressed and finely minced
$3/4$ tsp ground cinnamon
1 tsp poultry seasoning
Unrefined natural sea salt to taste (optional)

Combine broth, 1 tsp oil, and seasonings to make marinade.
Add the chicken breasts, forking the chicken several times to let
the marinade soak in. Put the chicken in the refrigerator to
marinate for at least 15–30 minutes. Preheat oven to 350
degrees. Meanwhile, remove chicken from the marinade, heat 2
tsp oil on medium heat, and brown the chicken breasts on both
sides. Place the chicken in a baking dish, drizzle half the marinade (including pieces of ginger and garlic) on top and bake for
15 minutes. After 15 minutes, pour additional marinade on top
and bake for 15–20 minutes more. Sprinkle entire dish lightly
with sea salt before serving. Serves 4.

TIPS FOR FOLLOWING
THE ENERGY-REVITALIZING DIET AT HOME

Because the Energy-Revitalizing Diet goes against most standard
nutritional advice given out today, sticking to it may require teaching

yourself some new food-preparation and eating habits. Here are some practical suggestions for making the diet easier for you to follow at home:

- Make sure to have some protein for breakfast—and be creative with your choices. Eggs are a great protein- and zinc-rich way to begin the day, but eating eggs over and over again can become monotonous fast. Other traditional American breakfast foods—cereal, toast, bagels, muffins, and pancakes—aren't good choices because they're low in zinc and protein and high in carbohydrates. To get the protein you need at breakfast—protein that will improve your energy and enhance copper detoxification—you may need to break through the bonds of conventional fare. Try occasionally having chicken and brown rice for breakfast, for example, or finishing off any lunch or dinner leftovers you have in the refrigerator.
- Plan ahead. If you wait to think about what to eat until you're already famished, chances are you'll grab anything you can find for quick energy. Remember that ready-to-eat convenience foods—whether they're zinc-depleted sugar or white-flour products, high-copper nuts, or high-calcium, high-fat cheese foods—all contribute to copper buildup. The foods that are most beneficial to your recovery—those high in unprocessed, zinc-rich animal protein—require some preparation. Make sure to have eggs, poultry, and lean meats on hand in your refrigerator and freezer, and schedule the time necessary to prepare these foods. Make it easy on yourself, though: keep meals as simple as possible.
- When you have time, particularly on weekends, make more food than you plan to eat in one sitting. That way you can have leftovers later in the week when you're too busy to cook from scratch. Try roasting a chicken, turkey, or beef or lamb roast, for example, and saving extra meat for other meals. These meats are all good cold on salads, or they can be added to soups or reheated and used creatively for future meals. Planning and preparing some food ahead of time makes following the diet much easier.
- Keep zinc-rich protein foods such as cooked meats, hard-boiled eggs, pumpkin seeds, and Pumpkorn—along with veggie sticks or fruit—on hand to have as snacks. Keep undesirable snacks—items

such as high-copper nuts or zinc-depleted crackers and cookies—out of your house so that you won't be tempted by them.

- Be gentle with yourself while making these diet changes. Going against standard nutritional advice and learning to eat the low-copper, high-zinc way may take time. Keep reminding yourself that increasing your intake of zinc and protein and avoiding high-copper foods will slowly but surely facilitate reversal of copper overload so that you can regain your energy. To help you reinforce these ideas, you might want to put the following note on your fridge:

Control copper.
Think zinc.
Pay more attention to protein.
Copper-and-zinc balance leads to better *energy*.

TIPS FOR FOLLOWING THE ENERGY-REVITALIZING DIET WHEN EATING OUT

More and more of us are eating many of our meals in restaurants. Most restaurants offer entrées that contain zinc-rich animal protein, so eating out on the Energy-Revitalizing Diet can be easier than eating in, providing you choose the right selections. The following are tips for helping you make the healthiest low-copper, high-zinc choices while eating out in a variety of different restaurant settings:

- In American-style and hotel restaurants, steer clear of copper-rich shellfish and liver; instead, stick with traditional, homespun meals like roast chicken or turkey or pot roast, choosing vegetables or a small baked potato for your side dish. Though fish is low in zinc, it can be a good protein choice for variety when eating out, particularly if you don't cook fish at home (which seems to be the case with many of my clients). If the menu offers mostly burgers and sandwiches, politely ask to have the meat or chicken served with a salad or veggies instead of a bun.
- If you go to a seafood restaurant, order fish—most any type of fish—but *not* shellfish. Although others who are dining with you

may partake of extremely high-copper foods such as oysters and lobster, remind yourself that these foods aren't good for you.

- If you eat Italian, forgo the pasta and bread and the shrimp or squid selections, choosing instead deliciously prepared veal, chicken, or fish with garlic and fresh herbs. Add a leafy green Italian salad and a medley of flavorful sautéed vegetables or a steamed artichoke, and you have a well-balanced meal. A choice that's always nice for lunch is a grilled chicken Caesar salad without the croutons.

- If you like to eat in Greek or Middle Eastern restaurants, many zinc-rich choices await you. These include roast leg of lamb, chicken Athenian, souvlaki (meat- or chicken-vegetable kabobs), gyros, and broiled lamb chops. If you prefer something lighter, try fish and a traditional Greek salad or Greek egg-lemon soup.

- In Chinese restaurants, avoid tofu and seafood dishes and opt for beef or chicken stir-fry with a variety of vegetables (but no mushrooms or nuts). Make sure the entrées you choose aren't served with a soy- or sugar-based sauce; sweet-and-sour, plum, and hoisin sauces should all be avoided.

- If you go to a Japanese restaurant, choose hibachi-style beef or chicken, but be careful of the many sauces that contain soy. Ask your server if your meal can be prepared without the sauce; most Japanese restaurants are more than happy to do this.

- In French and Continental restaurants, your best bets are poultry (such as *poulet aux fines herbes*—roast chicken with herbs), lamb, beef, or game meats or game birds. Poached salmon and other fish are less desirable because they're lower in zinc, but they're still good choices. Remember that mushroom dishes, liver-based foods (such as pâté de foie gras), seafood dishes (such as oyster stew or bouillabaisse), and desserts made with chocolate are all high in copper and should be avoided.

- When you're in the mood for Mexican food, avoid large amounts of high-calcium cheese and copper-rich beans. You're better off with zinc-rich protein choices—for example, chicken or beef fajitas, a chicken or beef taco salad, or grilled chicken or beef tacos. Fish prepared Veracruz style (with tomatoes, peppers, and onions) is a nice choice if you have trouble digesting protein and fat.

- When you go out for Indian food, look for meals prepared with high-zinc chicken or lamb. Good choices include chicken or lamb tandoori, korma, or kabobs. Avoid dishes that contain nuts, mushrooms, and dried fruits such as raisins.
- If you go to a natural-food restaurant, pass on meals that are vegetarian and choose those that contain some animal protein—fish, eggs, or poultry. This may sound like odd advice to those of us who have heard accolades about vegetarian eating, but it's exactly what you need to do to overcome copper overload. Be careful not to eat many zinc-depleting whole grains, especially whole-wheat products, in these restaurants.
- If you're eating on the run, look for fast-food outlets that offer health-conscious choices such as rotisserie-cooked chicken and turkey. Good side dishes to accompany the poultry at these restaurants include steamed, stewed, or baked vegetables, green salads, roasted red potatoes, or cooked sweet potatoes. Large salads or serve-yourself salad bars also are good choices if they contain some type of protein—hard-boiled egg, chicken, turkey, or tuna, perhaps—in addition to the greens. Avoid hamburger joints that serve greasy food, since fats are hard for those with copper overload to digest.
- If you're traveling or expect to have a delayed meal, take pumpkin seeds or Pumpkorn in your pocket or purse. These zinc-rich minimeals keep well wherever you go, are easy to carry, and are ready to eat when you need them.

PERSONALIZING THE ENERGY-REVITALIZING DIET

The basic Energy-Revitalizing Diet is a good place to start for those with copper overload, but as with all formula diets, it needs to be personalized according to the individual. I'm a firm believer that one diet simply can't be right for everyone. Although all individuals who have copper overload share the common bond of copper excess, each person's biochemistry differs dramatically in numerous ways. It's important, therefore, that you modify the Energy-Revitalizing Diet so that it's custom-designed for *you*. Consider the following factors as you make your modifications:

Copper Status

Each individual with copper excess differs in the degree of copper imbalance he or she has. Some of us have only a recent, mild case, while others have a more serious case that's been building for years.

The Energy-Revitalizing Diet was developed for people who have what I call "garden-variety" copper overload—typically, individuals who give six to eight affirmative answers on the copper overload questionnaire included in Chapter 7. If you have a less or more severe case of copper overload, it's best to modify your diet as outlined below:

- If you answered yes to nine to twelve questions (or if you show many of the signs of hidden copper imbalance—again, see Chapter 7—on a tissue mineral analysis), you may have a severe or long-standing case of copper overload. In that case, you may feel better completely avoiding red meats such as beef and lamb, as well as beans and pumpkin seeds. Red meats tend to be higher in fat than most fish and poultry and are therefore harder for those with copper overload to digest. Beans and pumpkin seeds—while good foods when eaten in moderation for most people with copper overload—contain some copper and generally should be avoided by those who have a more severe case.
- If you answered yes to three to five questions on the questionnaire (or if you have only slightly high copper levels on a tissue mineral analysis), you may be able to eat more red meats, pumpkin seeds, and beans than are shown in the sample weekly menu plan above. Try adding small amounts of these foods more frequently to your diet and see how you feel. If you become constipated, steer clear of these foods. In individuals with copper overload, constipation is usually a sign that such foods aren't being well digested.

Metabolism

Metabolism refers to the rate at which the body burns food for energy. Most people who have copper overload have a slow metabolism, so the Energy-Revitalizing Diet was designed with this in mind. With its emphasis on small, consistent intake of zinc and low-fat protein, this eating plan can jump-start a slow burner's sluggish metabolism, helping encourage the body to eliminate excess copper.

Fast burners—people who have a fast metabolism—don't often get copper overload, because they burn food quickly and eliminate toxins (including excess copper) efficiently. Occasionally, though, a fast burner who's exposed to a lot of external sources of copper or to a lot of stress (which, you'll recall, weakens the adrenal glands) will develop copper overload. You can determine whether you're a slow or a fast burner through tissue mineral analysis—remember: a buildup of minerals strongly suggests a slow metabolic rate—but your answer to the following simple question will give you a good indication: *Do you usually feel better—more calm, centered, and energetic—eating higher-fat protein sources such as red meats instead of lower-fat choices such as white-meat poultry and nonfatty fish?*

If your answer is yes, you're probably a fast burner. In that case, it's best to emphasize heavier, zinc-rich meats—foods such as beef, lamb, and dark-meat poultry—in your diet. If, on the other hand, these foods feel unpleasantly heavy and leave you constipated, avoid them until your copper imbalance improves.

Blood Type

Each of the four blood types (O, A, B, and AB) developed at a different stage in human evolution. At these various stages, our ancestors ate different combinations of foods. It's not surprising, then, that scientific research has revealed that each of the blood types contains antigens that react differently to the lectin proteins found in various foods. Because of these distinctions in development and protein reaction, the combinations and kinds of food people do best with often vary according to their blood type. Here are some suggestions for modifying the Energy-Revitalizing Diet according to *your* blood type:

- If you have type O blood, you may thrive on more lean red meats in your diet than the basic plan provides. Try adding lean cuts of beef, lamb, or game meats (such as buffalo, venison, and game birds), which are also rich in zinc. If constipation or digestive upset is a problem, though, stick with a preponderance of poultry and fish. Type O people usually don't do well with the more recent foods in the human diet—grains, legumes, and dairy products—so keep these foods to a minimum.
- If you have type A blood, avoid red meats; these tend to be poorly digested by type A people. You'll probably do better with a diet

that emphasizes eggs, poultry, fish, and pumpkin seeds as your primary protein sources.

- If you have type B blood, try to avoid chicken. It contains a lectin protein that's incompatible with your blood type and may cause subtle health problems that eventually lead to more serious problems over time. Eggs, turkey, and fish are always good choices for people of your blood type, and you can experiment with zinc-rich protein sources such as lamb, venison, rabbit, veal, buffalo, and pheasant.

- If you have type AB blood, you tend to have characteristics of both type A and type B folks. This means that, like type A people, you probably should avoid red meats; and, like type B people, you should avoid chicken. Turkey, eggs, fish, lamb, rabbit, and pheasant are all good choices for you.

Ancestry

Our ancestors originated in different parts of the world—Northern Europe, the Mediterranean area, North or South America, Asia, Africa. Each area had different local foods that were readily available, and our ancestors adapted biochemically to those native foods so that they could thrive. Since each of us carries some of that heritage from our ancestors in our genes, our ancestry may influence the types of foods we do best on. Research has shown, for example, that people who have ancestral heritages from northern areas (Irish, Celtic, Welsh, Scandinavian, Danish, British Columbian coastal native, or Eskimo backgrounds, for example) have an inherited need for more essential fatty acids (such as those found in cold-water fish like salmon) than people with other heritages. With this in mind, I often ask my clients to consider the type of diet their ancestors might have eaten and see if the foods found in that diet help them experience their best health. I encourage you to try this too, particularly if you belong exclusively to an ethnic group that has a specific diet.

Food Sensitivity

Individuals who have copper overload are prone to developing food sensitivities, because they usually have diminished adrenal gland function and difficulty digesting food. The foods most people with copper overload have trouble with are those high in copper—such as wheat, soy, yeast, mushrooms, nuts, and shellfish—which are avoided in the Energy-Revitalizing Diet. Other foods that can be problematic are legumes, which can be difficult to digest, and high-calcium foods such as dairy products. Both groups of foods are minimized in the diet I've outlined here. If you sense that legumes or dairy products (or any other foods, for that matter) bother you, completely eliminate them from your diet to see if your health improves. It's important to understand that even subtle reactions to foods can weaken adrenal function, contributing to copper buildup.

A Vegetarian Inclination

Individuals with copper overload often gravitate to vegetarian diets, because their condition makes it hard for them to digest meat. It's very difficult, however, to overcome copper overload while following a high-copper, low-zinc, low-protein vegetarian diet.

If you're a vegetarian, I strongly encourage you to begin slowly adding small amounts of animal protein, such as eggs or fish, to your diet. This will help to rev up both your metabolism and the copper detoxification process. Try taking hydrochloric acid and/or plant enzyme supplements with meals to help you digest and properly utilize the protein sources you eat. My clients often tell me these supplements are very helpful for preventing the heavy feeling that many vegetarians get after eating protein.

As your metabolism improves, gradually add more protein to your diet—especially more zinc-rich protein sources, such as chicken and turkey. Dairy products and soy foods, while good protein sources for some people, are best avoided if you have copper overload. Soy foods are very high in copper, and dairy products are very high in calcium and often in fat—all of which slow down the metabolism and exacerbate copper buildup.

I don't recommend a vegetarian diet for those with copper overload, but if you feel strongly about remaining on one, I have three suggestions:

- Deemphasize whole grains in your diet. They contain not only significant amounts of copper but also phytic acid, which interferes with the absorption of zinc. Most grain products also raise blood sugar levels in the same way sugar does (though to a lesser extent, of course), causing blood sugar fluctuations and energy highs and lows.

- Instead of grains, emphasize beans in your diet. They promote steadier blood sugar and energy levels and are a source of sulfur-rich amino acids that are needed for detoxification.

- Be sure to take supplements, especially supplements of zinc. (These will be covered in the next chapter.) Since a vegetarian diet is high in copper and low in zinc, you'll need to rely on supplements in higher amounts than do most people with copper overload.

Chapter Ten

The Complete Program for Conquering Copper Overload and Rebuilding Energy

The Energy-Revitalizing Diet is an essential part of conquering the fatigue that's associated with copper imbalance, but avoiding environmental copper, managing stress, and using the right nutrient supplements are equally important. My comprehensive program for reversing copper imbalance employs all of these components.

THE FOUR-PART APPROACH TO REVERSING COPPER OVERLOAD

To ensure the best chance of success, the program takes a four-part approach to recovery:

PART 1: Reduce exposure to copper.
PART 2: Use copper antagonists and chelating agents to inhibit copper absorption and to bind and remove excess copper from the body.
PART 3: Support optimal liver function and detoxification.
PART 4: Perhaps most important, enhance adrenal gland activity.

Let's take a look at each of these in depth.

Part 1: Reduce Exposure to Copper

If you have so much copper in your system that it's wreaking havoc with your energy, it only makes sense that you should reduce your exposure to copper to prevent further copper accumulation and aggravation of your condition. You can take several steps simultaneously to accomplish this. First, follow the Energy-Revitalizing Diet. With its avoidance of high-copper foods, this diet does much to prevent energy-draining copper buildup.

Second, supplement your diet with a *copper-free* multiple-vitamin/mineral supplement. Many people take a standard, over-the-counter multiple—most of which contain copper—to help meet nutritional needs, assuming that *any* supplement will enhance health. And yet for those who have copper overload, the copper found in multiples and other supplements contributes (sometimes dramatically) to their copper load and can aggravate their condition, lowering health and energy. Excess copper in the body can induce deficiencies of many other nutrients, so it's certainly a good idea to take a multiple-vitamin/mineral supplement. It's equally important, though, to take one that doesn't contain copper.

Copper-free multiples are hard to locate, because even in the natural-health industry, few people know about the problem of copper overload (meaning that most natural-product manufacturers don't make copper-free products). I became aware of this problem when I learned that I had copper overload many years ago. As a result of my frustration at not being able to find a product that met my needs, I worked with Uni Key Health Systems, a manufacturer of quality supplements, to develop a well-balanced, copper-free multiple. The supplement I developed, the Uni Key Female Multiple, is free of copper and specifically designed to meet the needs of women. I recommend it for all women who are tired and know or suspect that they have copper overload. To order this product or receive more information about it, call Uni Key at 800-888-4353.

There are a few other ways to minimize your exposure to copper. As I described in Chapter 8, it's important to determine whether you have high levels of copper in your water by using a water-testing kit; if you find that copper levels are high, take action to lessen this problem by investing in a filter that reduces copper or by finding a low-copper source of bottled water. If you opt for bottled water, remember that you're still bathing in copper-rich water. (You can determine the copper content of bottled water with the easy-to-use PurTest water-testing kit, or by writing the manufacturer of the particular brand of bottled water you're considering. Ask the manufacturer to send you a detailed chemical and mineral analysis of the water it's selling.)

Finally, be aware of any external sources of copper you're exposed to—anything from a copper IUD to some of the newer dental-filling compounds—and eliminate these whenever possible. This sometimes can make the difference between continuing to suffer from copper-induced fatigue and overcoming it for good.

Part 2: Use Copper Antagonists and Chelators

Many nutrients are antagonistic to copper and can either inhibit absorption of copper or bind copper and remove it from the body. When taken in supplement form, these copper-lowering nutrients can be used to assist the body in reversing copper overload. Zinc, for example, interferes with copper absorption and prevents copper accumulation. Other nutrients are helpful in different ways: manganese and iron displace copper from the liver; molybdenum and sulfur bind to copper in the intestine and greatly facilitate its excretion; and vitamin C chelates copper in the blood and facilitates its removal. Vitamin B-6 and niacin also help promote reversal of copper overload. You'll receive all these nutrients if you eat the range of foods I've included in the Energy-Revitalizing Diet, but the following food sources are especially high in one or more of these copper-antagonistic nutrients.

Zinc	Manganese
Chicken	Eggs
Turkey	Green leafy vegetables
Red meats	Pineapple
Wild game	Blueberries
Pumpkin seeds	

Iron	Molybdenum
Red meats	Dark-green vegetables
Spinach and other green leafy vegetables	Whole grains
Eggs	

Sulfur	Vitamin C
Eggs	Bell peppers
Meats	Broccoli
Garlic	Tomatoes
Onions	Citrus fruits
Hot chili peppers	Strawberries
Cruciferous vegetables such as broccoli, cauliflower, and brussels sprouts	Kiwi fruit

Vitamin B-6	Niacin
Fish	Turkey
Chicken	Chicken
Green leafy vegetables	Fish
Brown rice	Asparagus
Meats	

A well-balanced, nutrient-dense, omnivore diet can go a long way in combating copper overload, but nutrient supplements also are often needed. Specific amounts and combinations of nutrient supplements to conquer copper-induced fatigue should be individualized according to your symptoms, risk factors, diet, and tissue copper levels. To determine the most appropriate supplement program for you, it's best to have a tissue mineral analysis performed. All of the copper-antagonistic nutrients listed above typically are found in copper-free multiples, but most people who have moderate to severe cases of copper overload can benefit from taking additional amounts of zinc, manganese, vitamin B-6, and vitamin C along with a copper-free multiple.

Part 3: Support Liver Function and Detoxification

The liver regulates copper metabolism and is the major site of detoxification in the body; sluggish liver function typically is associated with copper buildup and underlies the fatigue that's associated with it. To encourage removal of stored copper from the body, it's essential that you support the liver's natural ability to detoxify. One of the main ways to do this is by eating foods and taking natural remedies that are rich in sulfur.

Sulfur is a mineral antagonistic to copper and all h
used by the body to form key amino acids, which
enzymes that are critical for detoxification. Sulfur also is nee
make protein-carrier molecules that pick up and transport copper in
the body. Recent research shows that the copper-binding protein,
metallothionine, cannot pick up the copper ion directly, but requires
the sulfur-based amino acid glutathione to act as an intermediary.
Several copper-overload experts believe this means that too little glutathione in the body (either from too little sulfur in the diet or from
exposure to chemicals that deplete the body's supply) contributes to
the development of copper overload. If we limit the body's exposure
to harmful chemicals and boost its supply of sulfur, however, we can
enhance detoxification and elimination of copper.

Food sources of sulfur are listed above. Since the Energy-Revitalizing
Diet includes a wide variety of these foods each day, following its guidelines can help increase sulfur status and enhance liver detoxification.
Sulfur-based natural remedies can provide additional support, especially
if sulfur-rich foods aren't on your list of favorites. One of the most effective supplements I've found for helping individuals recover from copper
overload is alpha lipoic acid. Although this sulfur-containing, vitamin-
like substance is unfamiliar to many Americans, lipoic acid has been
used effectively to treat heavy-metal toxicity in Europe. When taken in
amounts that can be obtained only through supplementation, lipoic
acid functions as a powerful chelator of heavy metals and as an antioxidant that may free up vitamins C and E and other antioxidants for other
tasks. It also acts as a co-enzyme that helps convert many food constituents (such as glucose and fatty acids) into energy. Given all these
functions, it isn't surprising that lipoic acid supplementation is one of
the best ways I've found to stimulate removal of stored copper from tissues and help restore energy in my clients. Lipoic acid supplementation
seems to be particularly effective for bringing deeply stored copper out
of the tissues in cases of hidden copper overload.

There are other remedies that also can be useful for supporting
liver function and detoxification. Black radish root, for example, is a
sulfur-containing herb that stimulates bile secretion, thereby encour-
aging elimination of excess copper from the system. Supplements of
sulfur-containing amino acids such as N-acetyl-cysteine and glutathione work in much the same way.

The liver detoxifies *all* toxins, not just excess copper. One of the best ways to enhance detoxification is to lighten the liver's workload by limiting the body's exposure to harmful chemicals. This means buying organically grown produce and organically raised meats whenever possible, as well as limiting exposure to other unnecessary chemicals—from household cleaners to pesticides used in the home or office.

Part 4: Boost Adrenal Function

Adrenal gland insufficiency is probably the most important contributing factor to copper overload and fatigue. As you'll recall from Chapter 5, the adrenals work together with the liver to facilitate proper copper transportation and utilization, as well as elimination of the excess. This means that to promote recovery from copper overload, taking steps to boost adrenal function is just as important as enhancing the liver's ability to detoxify. One important way to rejuvenate the adrenals is to lighten our stress load; another important strategy is to arm the adrenals with the nutrients they need to function optimally. Let's look at each of these in turn.

Boosting Adrenal Function Through Stress Reduction. We've already established that adrenal gland insufficiency is a prime determinant of copper overload and fatigue. But what causes that insufficiency? More often than not it's stress. Learning to lighten your stress load is therefore an absolute necessity as you attempt to rebuild energy and conquer fatigue and copper overload.

Remember that stress takes many forms. Some forms are physical (such as the stress most people feel from overwork or lack of sleep), and some are emotional. The stressors in this latter category are unique to each one of us. Something that evokes feelings of stress in one individual—driving a car, for example—might not affect another. To manage stress effectively, it's important to determine which things are particularly stressful to you and find creative ways to cope with the stressors you can't avoid. The following are my top suggestions for lessening stress and improving adrenal function:

1. Simplify your life. Remind yourself that your energy is needed right now to help your body heal from copper overload. Cut back on social activities and obligations that create stress and rob you of energy.

2. Do light to moderate exercise. Physical activity typically lessens stress, but it's important not to push yourself so far that you further deplete adrenal energy. Exercise at the level that feels best to you, even if that's only a short walk.

3. Take control of your life and your time, and don't blame others for your problems. Instead, learn to express yourself and tell others close to you what you really want and need from them. Make it a point not to take on extra responsibilities you'd rather not do (and will later resent).

4. Break the worry habit. Continually remind yourself that worrying won't change what's happening in your life, but the distress you feel from it will take its toll on your body's ability to overcome copper overload and regain energy.

5. Set priorities and stick with them. Save your energy for things that are important or rewarding to you. Fill your life with as many things as possible that give you pleasure and promote positive feelings.

6. Develop good sleeping habits, and take some time each day for rest and relaxation. Take frequent breaks from stress by doing whatever works best to lighten your stress load—whether that's reading comic books, listening to music, stretching, doing deep breathing, meditating, or talking to a trusted friend.

Strengthening Adrenal Function Through Supplements. Adrenal-enhancing nutrients include Vitamin C and the B-complex vitamins. Known as "antistress" vitamins, these nutrients are needed in high amounts—and are used up quickly—during periods of stress. Pantothenic acid (or vitamin B-5), is especially noteworthy for helping improve adrenal function: many adrenal hormones can't be manufactured without this nutrient. Moderate amounts of protein and fat in the diet also are necessary for healthy adrenal function: protein and fat provide the building blocks needed to make hormones that allow the body to cope with stress and that signal the liver to use and eliminate copper properly.

The Energy-Revitalizing Diet supplies a good range of all the nutrients needed for adrenal function. However, people who have weak adrenal function or are very stressed may benefit from taking more of these nutrients in supplemental form. Supplemental amounts of vitamin C as high as 3,000 milligrams are not excessive during times of chronic stress. A B-complex supplement (one that supplies at least 50 milligrams of each of the major B vitamins) also is helpful, and pantothenic acid in amounts of 100 milligrams extra each day can give a big boost to sluggish adrenal function. One formula I've found to be particularly helpful for those with fatigue and adrenal insufficiency or adrenal burnout is the Uni Key Adrenal Formula from Uni Key (800-888-4353). It contains not only pantothenic acid and vitamin C, but also bovine adrenal glandular tissue, an extract from animal adrenal glands that carries the DNA/RNA blueprint of the adrenal gland. Many of my copper overload clients who experience a lot of stress have found that providing potent nutrition for their worn-out adrenal glands is one of the most critical steps for recovering from copper overload and fatigue.

PUTTING YOUR SUPPLEMENT PROGRAM TOGETHER

A supplement program that's personalized according to an individual's symptoms, risk factors, and tissue copper levels always works best. Here are some guidelines to help you customize the best supplement program for you:

1. *If you know or strongly suspect that you have copper overload,* take a copper-free multiple to help protect against nutrient insufficiencies. A copper-free multiple is the foundation on which everyone with copper overload should build. See Appendix C for a listing of the nutrient amounts I recommend in a multiple for those with this condition. If you have a mild case of copper overload (that is, if you answered yes to three to five questions on the copper overload questionnaire found in Chapter 7), you'll probably need only to follow the Energy-Revitalizing Diet and take a copper-free multiple to balance copper levels in your system.

2. *If you have a moderate to severe case of copper overload* (that is, if you answered yes to six or more questions on the questionnaire, or if you have very high levels of copper or many signs of hidden copper imbalance on a tissue mineral analysis), you'll need a little extra help to facilitate removal of the stored copper from your body. Try taking the following amounts of individual supplements daily, in addition to a copper-free multiple:

Zinc	10–25 mg
Manganese	5–15 mg
Vitamin B-6	50–200 mg
Vitamin C	500–3,000 mg

It's important to note that while moderate amounts of copper-antagonistic nutrients are helpful for detoxification, too much of these nutrients can pull copper out of tissues too fast, sometimes causing uncomfortable symptoms. Read the labels of all supplements you're considering and be careful not to exceed a combined total of 50 milligrams daily for zinc, 30 milligrams for manganese, 300 milligrams for vitamin B-6, and 5,000 milligrams for vitamin C (unless you're working with a practitioner trained in treating copper overload who's monitoring your condition and advises you to do so).

3. *If you have a moderate to severe case of copper overload and suspect sluggish liver function,* try boosting your sulfur reserves with a daily dose of 50 to 150 milligrams of alpha lipoic acid, *or* 100 to 300 milligrams of black radish root, *or* 200 to 500 milligrams of N-acetyl-cysteine twice a day, and 50 to 150 milligrams of reduced glutathione.

4. *If you've been exposed to external sources of copper, such as a copper IUD or dental fillings that contain copper,* follow suggestions 1, 2, and 3 (above). To combat the copper burden you've been subjected to, strictly avoid copper in supplements and take extra amounts of zinc, manganese, vitamin B-6, vitamin C,

and lipoic acid to promote removal of stored copper from the system.

5. *If you take the birth control pill,* the same advice applies. Because the pill raises copper levels in the blood, extra amounts of copper antagonists are needed. The pill also tends to make the elimination of toxins from the liver sluggish, so sulfur-based remedies (such as alpha lipoic acid) that help detoxification are recommended.

6. *If you're under a lot of stress or suspect that you have adrenal insufficiency or adrenal burnout,* give your adrenals a nutrient boost with a B-50 complex, an extra 100 milligrams of pantothenic acid, raw bovine adrenal glandular tissue (200–600 milligrams), and up to 3,000 milligrams of vitamin C. (Be sure not to consume more than 5,000 milligrams total vitamin C—that is, in all your supplements combined—each day.)

7. *If you're a vegetarian and feel strongly about remaining one,* supplemental zinc is a must for your recovery. Be sure to take a copper-free multiple that contains vitamin B-12 as well as a supplemental zinc total of between 25 and 50 milligrams per day.

8. *To meet your needs for essential fatty acids (EFAs),* try to eat cold-water fish a few times a week or drizzle small amounts of flaxseed oil on your foods. Individuals with copper overload tend to be low in EFAs; and because of copper-induced zinc and vitamin B-6 deficiencies, their systems have trouble converting EFAs to prostaglandins, which help regulate many functions in the body, including hormonal balance. If you don't eat much cold-water fish or use flaxseed oil, consider taking supplements of evening primrose oil (four to six 500-milligram softgels daily) and fish oil (two softgels daily containing 180 milligrams EPA and 120 milligrams DHA). This is especially helpful when premenstrual syndrome or skin problems (such as dry skin or psoriasis) are involved.

Lastly, when using supplements to help reverse copper overload, keep in mind a few basics:

- Always take supplements with food. Nutrient supplements taken on an empty stomach can result in gastrointestinal upset and nausea. Furthermore, the nutrients in supplements are absorbed better when taken with food.
- Avoid taking zinc supplements at the same time you eat a high-fiber food, particularly a high-grain meal. The insoluble fiber and phytic acid in whole grains reduce zinc absorption.
- When using long-term, high-zinc therapy (more than 45 milligrams per day) to help reverse copper overload, it's a good idea to have your doctor monitor your LDL and HDL cholesterol levels: excessive amounts of zinc can cause "bad" (LDL) cholesterol levels to rise and "good" (HDL) cholesterol levels to drop. If significant unfavorable alterations in your LDL and HDL cholesterol levels occur, reduce the amount of zinc you take.

COPPER DUMPS: POTHOLES ON THE ROAD TO RECOVERY

Using supplements appropriately helps promote recovery from copper-induced fatigue, but anyone who's ever healed from anything can appreciate that healing is an up-and-down process. If you sprain your ankle, for example, the ankle might improve amazingly well for a couple of weeks; then, just when you think you can put on your dancing shoes again, the ankle begins to throb and swell. This is the zigzag nature of healing.

This up-and-down process can also occur when people attempt to reverse copper overload and the fatigue and other symptoms that come with it. The Energy-Revitalizing Diet and supplement program presented here are designed to stimulate removal of copper stored in tissues, but they can't guarantee a smooth road to success. Occasionally the detoxification process occurs so fast that it results in temporary, unpleasant symptoms. These are called *copper dumps* or *copper reactions*.

During copper dumps, copper is eliminated from storage depots in the tissues and released into the blood, causing blood levels of copper to rise. If copper is released more quickly than the liver can eliminate it, copper levels in the blood rise *too* high, resulting in a mild version of copper poisoning. Typical copper-dump symptoms include nausea and other digestive disorders, anxiety, mental racing and hyperactivity, irritability, emotional volatility, headaches, insomnia, skin rashes, and mild flulike symptoms.

Copper-dump symptoms can be distressing and frustrating for individuals combating copper overload—especially for those who weren't aware that such side effects could occur. If individuals with copper overload don't mentally prepare themselves for the possibility of dumps, they tend to become discouraged or frustrated if such symptoms do develop. Some people take copper dumps as signs that the copper-control program isn't working, and they abandon treatment.

If you take steps to reverse copper overload and find yourself experiencing copper-dump symptoms, keep in mind several things. First, these symptoms are temporary, usually lasting only a day or two. Furthermore, copper-dump symptoms are signs that the excess copper in your tissues— the source of your fatigue—is being corrected. While these symptoms can be uncomfortable, they should be welcomed as indicators that the underlying problem behind your health concerns is being addressed and that true healing is taking place. Bear in mind that the severity of copper dumps and the length of time it takes the body to bring copper levels into the optimal range are individual matters. Some people hardly notice copper dumps and get over copper overload quickly. Others—generally those with more long-standing copper imbalance—go through periods of feeling well followed by periods in which they experience uncomfortable copper-dump symptoms many times before their condition is corrected.

When healing from copper overload, be prepared for mild healing discomfort from time to time. If the copper-dump symptoms you experience become too distressing, however, there are several ways to deal with them. Individuals with copper overload typically learn through experience which methods work best for them. You can find your own best method from among the following suggestions:

- Because stress often triggers copper dumps, make a special effort at this time to reduce stressors and to cope creatively with the stress you can't avoid. Keep life simple, get moderate exercise, take

control over your life, limit your worrying to what' [...]
(and honor) priorities, and schedule adequate rest.

- Make sure you're getting enough vitamin B-6, vitamin [...] [...]c. Many of the symptoms associated with copper dumps a[...] related to a copper-induced deficiency in these nutrients. When vitamin B-6, vitamin C, and zinc reserves are adequate, excess copper released into the bloodstream can be contained (and copper-dump symptoms can thereby largely be prevented).

- If the previous suggestion doesn't work for you, cut back on the amounts of supplements you're taking for a day or two. This typically slows down elimination of copper from the tissues, allowing copper-dump symptoms to subside.

- Another strategy is to temporarily add more calcium or dairy foods (such as low-fat cheese) to your diet. This tends to slow both the metabolism and the elimination of copper. Once your uncomfortable symptoms lift, however, you should return to the original Energy-Revitalizing Diet and steer clear of most high-calcium foods.

- Try taking 100 milligrams of molybdenum, a mineral that helps clear excess copper out of the bloodstream. It can be helpful in relieving some of the disagreeable reactions that sometimes result from copper elimination.

- If you find yourself feeling extremely emotional, anxious, or panicky for no apparent reason, try to employ logic: remind yourself that these are symptoms arising from high copper levels and imbalanced body chemistry. To help take the edge off emotionality until body chemistry improves, experiment with Bach flower remedies or with homeopathic remedies developed for nervousness or depression. Another strategy that's proved helpful for some of my clients is to take 400 milligrams of magnesium, a mineral that has relaxing properties, for a day or two.

A FINAL WORD ON GETTING WELL

The program for conquering copper overload outlined in this chapter addresses copper overload from all angles. By reducing exposure to copper, using supplements of copper-antagonistic nutrients, supporting liver function and detoxification, enhancing adrenal activity, and reducing stress, the program addresses *all* cases of copper overload, no matter what the individual contributing factors. Many people will feel better quickly after beginning the copper-control program; those with more severe copper overload will need to follow the plan for several months before seeing improvements in energy and well-being.

It's important to understand that the program outlined in this chapter is *not* a quick-fix, Band-Aid treatment for fatigue. It gets to the root of the problem, strengthening the body so that it can slowly but surely correct copper imbalance. Since most cases of copper imbalance and the fatigue that comes with it develop gradually over a period of many years, individuals with copper overload shouldn't expect to regain energy overnight. How long it takes the body to rebuild energy varies depending on many factors, including how severe the overload is and how long it's been developing.

If you've had copper-related fatigue and other health problems for a long time, you're probably impatient to see results, but I encourage you to be patient and adopt a long-term approach to regaining your health. In my experience working with clients, I've noted that the more persistent and consistent individuals are in following the copper-control program, the more surely their copper levels normalize. And when copper levels in the body normalize, the energy-dampening burden the body has been carrying lifts, and health and vitality return.

How do you know when you've completely recovered from copper overload? Tissue mineral analysis can tell you. The best answer, though, lies in how you feel. If you feel energetic, healthy, and centered for at least three months without slipping—and if you consistently score low on the copper overload questionnaire—you've officially conquered copper overload.

Once you've reached that point, congratulations are in order! Your next step is to embark on a preventive program that maintains high energy and *keeps* you well.

Chapter Eleven

Maintaining High Energy and Preventing Future Copper Overload

Maintaining health and vitality after copper overload is an ongoing balancing act. Individuals who've suffered from copper overload and its attendant fatigue remain at risk for that condition. Chances are they'll need to guard against copper overload all their life to protect their health and conserve their energy. This predisposition toward a certain condition isn't unique to those with copper overload: we all incline more toward one or two health problems than to others. If you've had copper overload, then, you know you're still susceptible to the condition. This doesn't mean that you're destined to suffer from copper overload, only that you need to be savvy to maintain a high energy level and prevent recurrence of copper excess.

According to the late Paul C. Eck, who spent decades specializing in the study of copper overload, certain people are "copper personalities"—individuals who are sensitive, emotional, bright, and creative. They tend naturally to carry higher levels of copper in the body, which is good in many ways: the copper helps stimulate or accentuate innovative thinking, emotional warmth, and artistic ability. However, because individuals with copper personalities are very sensitive, they're susceptible to stress-induced anxiety and are much more prone than other people to *re*develop copper overload.

If you fit the description of the copper personality, appreciate yourself for the kind of person you are—a talented but finely tuned individual. Understand that the tendency toward high copper has its upside—copper helps promote many valuable qualities—but it also means that you need to be especially diligent at managing stress effectively and keeping copper levels in check to prevent copper-induced fatigue and other health problems.

To protect the health and energy you've worked so hard to regain, you need to resolve not to go back to the bad health habits that caused you to develop copper overload in the first place. Instead, you need to adopt a maintenance plan—a more lenient, flexible version of the energy-revitalizing program described in earlier chapters. This means fine-tuning your savvy about copper and zinc, regularly monitoring your symptoms and risk factors with periodic checkups, and adjusting your diet and supplement program accordingly.

FINE-TUNING YOUR SAVVY

In order to overcome copper overload and rebuild your energy, you had to learn to look at nutrition and environment in a new way—through copper-colored glasses. You learned that stress, birth control pills, copper IUDs, many dental-filling compounds, drugs, chemicals, and plant protein–based meals all contribute to copper overload. You also learned that the best ways to keep zinc levels in healthy ranges are to eat land-based animal protein; avoid zinc-zappers such as alcohol, coffee, and sugar; take appropriate amounts of supplemental zinc when needed; and manage stress effectively.

To maintain your energy after copper overload, you must not only recall all that information but build on it with additional input from your own body. Keeping in mind what you know about copper and zinc, you can begin now to *gradually* loosen the reins on copper in your diet. Start by adding small amounts of copper-containing foods to your diet every few days. If you continue to feel healthy and energetic and don't experience any unusual symptoms, try adding a little more of these foods a little more often. Continue to do this with a variety of copper-rich foods. Each step of the way, ask yourself how you're feeling. If you begin to feel out of balance—physically fatigued but mentally or emotionally hyperactive and anxious—you've probably tipped the scales too far in favor of copper. It's then time to be stricter with your diet again, cutting back on copper and emphasizing zinc. Be sure to watch out for mood swings and cravings for more copper-rich foods. These are usually signs that your body isn't ready for as much copper in your diet as it's getting. Gradually, through trial and error, you'll find the right combinations and amounts of zinc- and copper-rich foods to keep you both energized and centered.

Many Americans are familiar with the concept of balancing carbohydrates, protein, and fat in the diet—a balancing act that differs from person to person—in order to maintain high energy levels. This same concept can be applied to copper and zinc in the diet. Through experimentation with your diet, you can use the signals your body gives you to keep copper and zinc in healthy ranges and avoid a redevelopment of copper overload and subsequent diminishment of energy. Each one of us probably has a different balance of copper and zinc that we do best on, but it's safe to say that most of us need more zinc in our diets than we presently get. Recent research shows that our distant ancestors consumed an average of 43 milligrams of zinc per day, yet most of us consume only 5 to 14 milligrams per day. I believe that people generally need at least two zinc-rich meals a day to keep healthy, although many individuals prone to copper overload seem to do best when they have small amounts of zinc-rich foods several times throughout the day.

The need for zinc is especially strong when we're stressed. As you'll recall, stress is a big-time drainer of both zinc and energy, and when zinc levels drop and copper levels rise, physical exhaustion and emotional anxiety can result. To keep balanced during stress, we need to compensate by tipping the scales in favor of zinc. Many of my clients have told me that when they do this, they remain energetic and emotionally centered even in pressure-filled situations.

Learning to manage stress effectively is a critical part of maintaining health and high energy levels. You may remember from earlier chapters that excessive stress is the number-one factor for many people in loss of energy. In this day and age, most of us are exposed to countless stressful situations, but we can do two things to combat stress's energy-draining effects. The first is to learn to change our attitude and control our reactions to those situations. The second is to take some time out after extremely stressful periods to relax, take good care of ourselves, and allow the adrenals to rejuvenate. When the adrenals are allowed to recharge, they help give us extra get-up-and-go when we need it. This second suggestion involves a skill all individuals prone to copper overload need to develop into a fine art.

MONITORING YOUR STATUS WITH PERIODIC CHECKUPS

Like any maintenance plan, your efforts to maintain health and energy after copper overload require you to initiate regular checkups. Just as you take your car to a mechanic for periodic checkups to prevent the development of major problems, so too should you check yourself out. A number of tests, as you'll see below, can be helpful. Depending on the results of these tests, you can take appropriate action to keep copper and zinc levels from getting out of line.

Hormone Testing

You'll recall from Chapter 6 that there's a close relationship between copper and estrogen levels in the body, and between zinc and progesterone. Given that connection, keeping tabs on estrogen and progesterone levels in the body can give valuable information about one's copper and zinc status.

The measuring of estrogen and progesterone levels can be done through a blood or urine test at your doctor's office. Another less expensive, noninvasive, and more convenient method for determining hormone levels is a saliva test. This can be conducted on your own, in the privacy of your home. If you'd like to determine your hormone levels this way, you can order saliva tests for estrogen and progesterone through Uni Key. (See Salivary Hormone Testing in the Resources section of this book.)

Whether you have a blood, urine, or saliva test taken, if you find your estrogen levels high and your progesterone levels low, you should suspect that copper levels in your body are getting out of balance with zinc. You can use the results of estrogen and progesterone tests to give you clues as to how to adjust your diet and nutrition supplements to promote continued health and energy.

Tissue Mineral Analysis

As explained in Chapter 7, tissue mineral analysis provides a unique reading of what occurs, metabolically speaking, in the cells (or energy-manufacturing centers) of the body over a three-month period. If you send a sample of hair in for analysis from time to time, you can obtain periodic readings of your tissue copper, zinc, and other mineral levels. This information is invaluable for helping you fine-tune your supplement program for optimal energy and well-being. It's particularly helpful for knowing whether you should supplement with copper or not.

Most of this book has focused on *avoiding* copper if you have copper overload, but it's important to remember that *some* copper is needed for optimal energy production. Since both too much and too little copper can cause fatigue, tissue mineral analysis is extremely helpful; it serves as a crystal ball through which you can examine your copper and zinc levels. These readings can help you determine if you should supplement with copper (or zinc) after regaining your energy, and they can indicate trends toward health problems that may be developing slowly without your knowledge. I recommend tissue mineral analysis at least once or twice a year as a way to receive information that you can use to keep your energy levels consistently high.

The Copper Overload Questionnaire

The easiest and quickest way to check your copper status is to refer back every few months to the copper overload questionnaire found in Chapter 7. The questionnaire is specifically designed to assess copper personality traits, symptoms, and risk factors that are indicative of copper overload. Generally speaking, the more affirmative answers you have when you take the questionnaire, the more sick and tired you probably feel, and the more you suspect that copper overload is creeping back into the picture. The higher you score when taking the questionnaire, the more you need to take action: adopt a strict diet and supplement program to stop copper overload in its tracks and protect your health and energy before they deteriorate. The lower you score, on the other hand, the more lenient with your diet and supplements you can be.

MAINTAINING GOOD RESERVES OF NUTRIENTS

Optimal nutrition is at the heart of maintaining health, sustaining energy, and preventing disease—whether that disease be copper overload or any other health problem. The foods that provide us with the most nutrients are always *whole* foods—that is, foods in their natural state. As you learned in Chapter 4, whole foods and whole-food meals that are plant-based are high in copper and relatively low in zinc. These foods need to be limited in the diet of people who are trying to overcome copper overload, but most individuals on an energy-maintenance program *after* copper overload can enjoy vegetarian, macrobiotic, and other higher-copper, whole-food meals from time to time without a problem. This is especially true if they have high-zinc meals at other times throughout the day and/or take zinc supplements. Remember, though, that finding the exact combination of whole foods that promote health after copper overload is a delicate balancing act for each of us.

Maintaining good reserves of nutrients that are antagonistic to copper is one of the most important ways to help ensure that copper-induced fatigue doesn't redevelop. Individuals who are prone to copper overload need to be especially careful to maintain good reserves of three nutrients in particular: zinc, vitamin C, and vitamin B-6. The importance of zinc has been discussed repeatedly throughout this book, but high levels of vitamins C and B-6 are crucial as well. Adequate amounts of these nutrients on a day-to-day basis help prevent a recurrence of copper overload. Women especially don't get enough zinc, vitamin C, or vitamin B-6 in their diet, so it isn't surprising that many women suffer not only from fatigue but also from other health conditions associated with copper overload, including premenstrual tension, anxiety, depression, and low immunity. To keep these conditions from developing, most women can benefit from supplements that contain zinc, vitamin C, and vitamin B-6, especially during the premenstrual phase of their cycle, when copper and estrogen levels tend to be higher.

DEVELOPING A FLEXIBLE WELLNESS PROGRAM

The most important thing to watch out for in terms of protecting energy are insidious copper culprits—those that can either slowly add to your copper load or quickly leave you susceptible to copper buildup when received in large amounts. To refresh your memory, they're listed below:

INSIDIOUS COPPER CULPRITS

Water that contains high levels of copper
A copper IUD
Birth control pills and estrogen replacement therapy
Many of the newer dental-filling compounds
Overexposure to chemicals and certain drugs

Be sure to keep a watchful eye out for these health-eroding culprits; avoid them as much as possible to help ensure continued health and energy.

If you're regularly exposed to one or several of the culprits listed above, take preventive measures, adjusting your diet and supplement program accordingly. For example, if you use the pill as a method of birth control or to regulate your periods, be especially copper savvy and strict with your diet, and supplement that nutrition with extra amounts of vitamin B-6 and zinc to help counteract the pill's copper-raising effects. Doing this should help to minimize the increased risk of copper overload that people face when taking the pill. For some people, though, the pill simply isn't an option; those who are especially prone to copper overload generally aren't able to experience their best health and energy until they go off both the pill and the copper IUD.

If you're like most of my clients who've overcome copper-induced fatigue and regained wellness, you'll probably become inherently sensitive to the many factors that can throw copper and zinc levels off balance. You'll probably quickly sense environmental factors and foods that are wrong for you and intuitively learn to adjust your diet and supplement program according to the circumstances. By performing checkups periodically with the various tests mentioned above, you can add to this intuitive knowledge and individualize the right maintenance program for you.

Afterword

This book has introduced you to the connection between copper overload and fatigue, and it's touched on the copper connection to other common health problems. It contains both decades-old information and recent research. I have no doubt, however, that I've only scratched the surface of copper overload's impact on health. The truth is there's a lot we still don't know about copper metabolism. If you read any of the latest studies, you'll discover that's a consistent theme running throughout.

Modern medicine's understanding of copper overload is sketchy because most practitioners and researchers don't recognize subtle cases of copper toxicity as the common health problems that they are; therefore, little research is done in this area. Those researchers who are aware that copper can be a problem typically don't know how to test for high tissue copper levels. This means that much of the research exploring copper problems is either inaccurate or irrelevant. Most of what's known about copper overload is based on the clinical experience of practitioners such as myself—people who work with clients who have the condition.

I'm the first to acknowledge that there's a great need for more legitimate scientific research into the subject. I hope that this book will stimulate interest among the scientific community to conduct that research. Just as iron overload wasn't taken seriously until researchers joined the bandwagon of clinicians who saw the problem in their practices, I believe that copper overload will move from doctors' offices to laboratories. I predict that eventually—perhaps in a decade or so—copper overload will be recognized as a common cause of both fatigue and a variety of other health problems that don't respond well to standard medical and natural treatments.

Until that time, however, it's up to you to use the information presented in this book to your advantage. The information is controver-
sial, but cutting-edge health news always is. Having read this book,
you now know the latest on copper overload—and you know more
about the subject than most doctors. It's time to incorporate this new
knowledge into your life, using it to enjoy vibrant health and energy.

Appendix A

Examples of Copper Levels on Tissue Mineral Analysis Charts

As mentioned in Chapter 7, most doctors haven't been taught how to properly interpret tissue mineral analysis results to determine copper overload. The next several pages offer two direct and two hidden examples of copper excess, as shown through tissue mineral analysis.

Copper Overload Example 1 (Direct)

The following example shows both high tissue copper and a low zinc-to-copper ratio—two clear signs of copper overload. This tissue mineral analysis came from a female client who experienced copper-related fatigue, depression, and scoliosis.

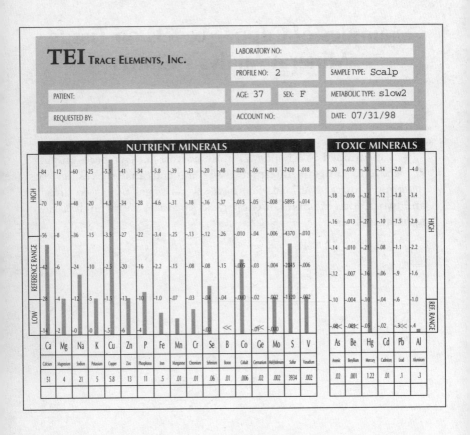

TEI TRACE ELEMENTS, INC.

LABORATORY NO:		
PROFILE NO: 2	SAMPLE TYPE: Scalp	
PATIENT:	AGE: 37	SEX: F	METABOLIC TYPE: slow2
REQUESTED BY:	ACCOUNT NO:	DATE: 07/31/98

NUTRIENT MINERALS

	Ca	Mg	Na	K	Cu	Zn	P	Fe	Mn	Cr	Se	B	Co	Ge	Mo	S	V
	Calcium	Magnesium	Sodium	Potassium	Copper	Zinc	Phosphorus	Iron	Manganese	Chromium	Selenium	Boron	Cobalt	Germanium	Molybdenum	Sulfur	Vanadium
	51	4	21	5	5.8	13	11	.5	.01	.01	.06	.01	.006	.02	.002	3934	.002

TOXIC MINERALS

	As	Be	Hg	Cd	Pb	Al
	Arsenic	Beryllium	Mercury	Cadmium	Lead	Aluminum
	.02	.001	1.22	.01	.1	.3

Copper Overload Example 2 (Direct)

The following is another example of copper excess and a low zinc-to-copper ratio. This chart belonged to a 54-year-old woman who had copper-related fatigue and dermatitis.

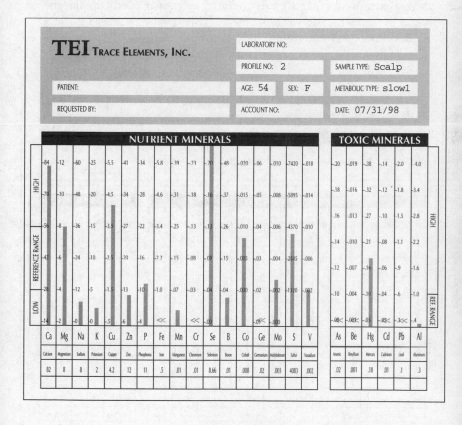

Copper Overload Example 3 (Hidden)

Here's an example of hidden copper excess. Even though the copper level is about normal, the very high calcium level and low zinc-to-copper ratio are indicators of an underlying copper overload situation that hasn't presented itself on the tissue mineral analysis yet. The female client whose hair was sampled for this analysis experienced several symptoms that are often related to copper overload—fatigue, yeast overgrowth, and viral infections. This is yet one more indicator to make the determination of hidden copper overload.

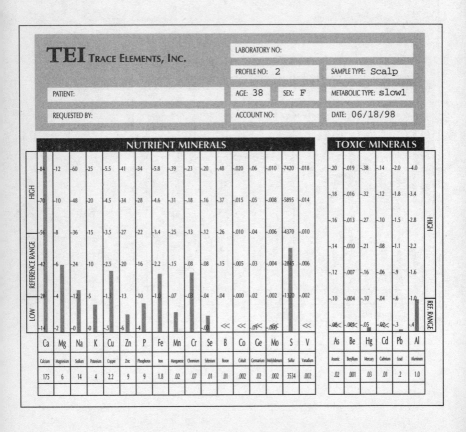

Copper Overload Example 4 (Hidden)

The following is another example of hidden copper overload. This chart belonged to a 41-year-old male who experienced fatigue, depression, and other symptoms of hypothyroidism—symptoms that also are associated with copper overload. Even though the copper level on the chart is low, the high calcium and high mercury levels both indicate the possibility of underlying copper excess.

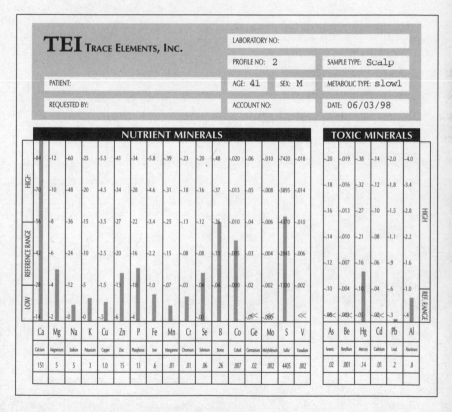

				TEI Trace Elements, Inc.							LABORATORY NO:					

PROFILE NO: 2   SAMPLE TYPE: Scalp

PATIENT: AGE: 41   SEX: M   METABOLIC TYPE: slow1

REQUESTED BY: ACCOUNT NO: DATE: 06/03/98

	Ca	Mg	Na	K	Cu	Zn	P	Fe	Mn	Cr	Se	B	Co	Ge	Mo	S	V
	Calcium	Magnesium	Sodium	Potassium	Copper	Zinc	Phosphorus	Iron	Manganese	Chromium	Selenium	Boron	Cobalt	Germanium	Molybdenum	Sulfur	Vanadium
	151	5	5	3	1.0	15	13	.6	.01	.01	.06	.26	.007	.02	.002	4405	.002

TOXIC MINERALS

As	Be	Hg	Cd	Pb	Al
Arsenic	Beryllium	Mercury	Cadmium	Lead	Aluminum
.02	.001	.14	.01	.2	.8

These tissue mineral analysis charts and case descriptions are reprinted courtesy of Trace Elements, Inc., a federally licensed tissue mineral analysis laboratory in Addison, Texas.

Appendix B

Testing Your Water with a Home Water-Testing Kit

The only way to know for sure whether your water is contributing to copper buildup and thereby sabotaging your ability to sustain or regain energy is to test it. In the past, people had to go to the trouble and expense (up to several hundred dollars) of asking professional laboratories to do this. Fortunately, Donald R. Podrebarac, a consumer advocate and water industry expert, recently developed a series of easy, EPA-based, do-it-yourself water-testing products that allow users to quickly check levels of copper as well as other contaminants in whatever water they choose—whether it be tap water, filtered water, or bottled water.

The specific kit that allows you to test for copper in your water is called the PurTest Iron Hardness Plus. (It enables you to test for copper and iron as well as six other common contaminants or conditions.) This kit, available in many hardware and home-improvement stores, retails for about eight dollars, and the test is simple to conduct. All you have to do is fill the vial that's included in the kit with a sample of water, dip one test strip into the vial for 30 seconds with a constant back-and-forth motion, then remove the strip and match the color that develops on it to the color guide provided. If the color on your test strip matches or is darker than the color that indicates 1 ppm (part per million) of copper in water, the copper level in your water is probably contributing to or exacerbating your copper overload situation and fatigue. The EPA standard for excessive copper in water is 1.3 ppm, but several times in the past the EPA has established safe values of other contaminants at levels that turned out to be too high. For individuals with high tissue copper levels, I believe it's prudent to be more cautious about copper levels in water than the EPA now advocates.

A wide variety of water filters can reduce copper levels in the water, but the type of filter that works best depends on the source of the excess copper. The water treatment system I use is the Doulton ceramic water filter, which eliminates not only copper but also lead, chlorine, and pesticides; it also removes bacteria and parasites. For more information about the Doulton filter, call 800-888-4353. To learn more about what type of filter would be most effective for correcting the copper problem in your water, contact the American Water Service at 800-788-4825.

Appendix C

Recommended Amounts of Nutrients in a Copper-Free Multiple

If you have copper overload, I recommend a copper-free multiple, which can be hard to find. The following is the list of ingredients found in one day's dosage of the Uni Key Female Multiple, which I developed specifically for women who have copper-induced fatigue. If you're a male who has copper overload, look for a copper-free multiple that contains nutrients in approximately the same proportions, but choose one that's free of iron and that doesn't contain wild yam root and dong quai root.

Vitamin A	10,000 I.U.
Betacarotene	15,000 I.U.
Vitamin B-1	100 mg
Vitamin B-2	10 mg
Vitamin B-3 (niacinamide)	130 mg
Vitamin B-5 (pantothenic acid)	100 mg
Vitamin B-6 (PSP)	25 mg
Vitamin B-12	400 mcg
Folic acid	800 mcg
Choline	100 mg
Biotin	300 mcg
Vitamin C (calcium ascorbate)	1,000 mg
Vitamin E	400 I.U.

Calcium	250 mg
Magnesium	500 mg
Potassium	99 mg
Iron	15 mg
Zinc	5 mg
Manganese	20 mg
Iodine	150 mcg
Selenium	200 mcg
Boron	2 mg
Molybdenum	200 mcg
Chromium	200 mcg
Vanadyl Sulfate	200 mcg
Plant enzymes	
(amylase, protease, lipase, cellulase)	4,200 units
Wild yam extract (6%)	400 mg
Dong quai root	200 mg

Appendix D

Recommended Daily Allowances for Copper and Zinc

Recommended Daily Allowances for Copper

Infants	0.6 mg
Children Under 4 Years of Age	1.0 mg
Adults and Children 4 or More Years of Age	2.0 mg
Pregnant or Lactating Women	2.0 mg

Recommended Daily Allowances for Zinc

Infants	5 mg
Children Under 4 Years of Age	8 mg
Adults and Children 4 or More Years of Age	15 mg
Pregnant or Lactating Women	15 mg

Appendix E

Amounts of Copper and Zinc in Various Common Foods

The following is a list of the copper and zinc contents in various common foods found in *Nutrition Almanac*. The foods marked with an asterisk (*) contain zinc-inhibiting phytic acid. This means that the zinc they contain—even if it's a lot—isn't absorbed well.

	Quantity	mg Zinc	mg Copper
RDA for Adults		*15.00*	*2.00*
Breads			
Bagel	1	0.4	0.42
Rye bread	1 slice	0.3*	0.03
Cereals			
All-Bran	1 oz	3.7*	0.32
Bran, 100%	1/2 cup	2.5*	0.45
Bran Flakes, Kellogg's	3/4 cup	3.7*	0.21
Corn grits, cooked	1 cup	0.2	0.03
Fruit/Fibre (Mt. Trail)	1/2 cup	1.5	0.23
Golden Grahams	3/4 cup	0.3	0.23
Nutri-Grain, wheat	3/4 cup	3.7*	0.15

	Quantity	mg Zinc	mg Copper
Oatmeal, cooked	1 cup	1.2	0.13
Raisin Bran	1/2 cup	1.5	0.20
Rolled oats, dry	1 cup	2.5	0.28
Total	1 cup	0.8	0.14
Wheat Chex	2/3 cup	0.7	0.17
Wheat germ, toasted	1/4 cup	4.7*	0.18

Dairy Foods

Cheese

	Quantity	mg Zinc	mg Copper
Monterey jack	1 oz	0.9	0.01
Mozzarella, part skim	1 oz	0.8	0.01
Swiss	1 oz	1.1	0.04

Milk

	Quantity	mg Zinc	mg Copper
Goat	1 cup	0.7	0.10
Skim	1 cup	1.0	0.10
Soy	1 cup	0.5	0.29

Drinks

Alcoholic Beverages

	Quantity	mg Zinc	mg Copper
Beer	12 oz	0.1	0.30
Beer, lite	12 oz	0.1	0.09
Gin, rum, vodka, whiskey	1 oz	0.0	0.02
Wine, dessert	2 oz	0.0	0.03
Wine, red	3.5 oz	0.1	0.03
Wine, white	3.5 oz	0.1	0.03

Fruit Juices

	Quantity	mg Zinc	mg Copper
Apple juice	6 oz	0.1	0.02
Lemon juice	1 Tbsp	0.0	0.01
Lemonade *(frozen concentrate)*	6 oz	0.1	0.05
Lime juice	1 Tbsp	0.0	0.01
Orange juice	8 oz	0.1	0.11
Prune juice	8 oz	0.5	0.17

	Quantity	mg Zinc	mg Copper
Miscellaneous			
Coffee	6 oz	0.0	0.01
Coffee, flavored	6 oz	0.0	0.03
Cola	12 oz	0.1	0.10
Vegetable Juices			
Carrot juice	6 oz	0.3	0.09
Tomato juice	6 oz	0.3	0.18
V-8 juice	6 oz	0.4	0.40
Eggs			
Chicken, whole	1 large	0.7	0.10
Fish			
Abalone, fried	3 oz	0.8	0.19
Anchovies, canned, in oil	5	0.5	0.07
Clams, steamed	3 oz	2.3	0.59
Cod, baked	3 oz	0.5	0.03
Crab, moist-heat-cooked	3 oz	6.5	1.00
Crayfish, steamed	3 oz	1.4	0.48
Flatfish, baked	3 oz	0.5	0.02
Grouper, broiled	3 oz	0.4	0.04
Haddock, baked	3 oz	0.4	0.03
Halibut, baked	3 oz	0.5	0.03
Lobster, steamed	3 oz	2.5	1.70
Mackerel, baked	3 oz	0.8	0.08
Ocean perch, baked	3 oz	0.5	0.13
Perch, baked	3 oz	1.2	0.16
Pike, baked	3 oz	0.7	0.06
Salmon, poached	3 oz	0.4	0.06
Sardines, in oil	2	0.3	0.05
Shrimp, breaded, fried	3 oz	1.2	0.23
Snapper, baked	3 oz	0.4	0.04
Swordfish, baked	3 oz	1.3	0.14
Trout, rainbow, baked	3 oz	1.2	0.12
Tuna, water-packed	3 oz	0.4	0.01

	Quantity	mg Zinc	mg Copper
Flours			
Buckwheat	1 cup	3.5	0.70
Corn	1 cup	2.0	0.27
Peanut, defatted	1 cup	0.3	1.12
Rye, dark	1 cup	7.1*	0.96
Rye, light	1 cup	1.8*	0.30
Soy, defatted	1 cup	2.5*	4.10
Soy, full-fat	1 cup	3.3*	2.50
Soy, low-fat	1 cup	1.0*	4.50
Whole wheat	1 cup	2.9*	0.60
Grains and Grain Products			
Barley, pearl, cooked	1 cup	1.3	0.17
Brown rice, cooked	1 cup	1.2	0.20
Bulgur, cooked	1 cup	1.0	0.14
Macaroni, cooked	1 cup	0.7	0.14
Spaghetti, enriched, cooked	1 cup	0.7	0.14
Wheat bran	1 cup	5.6*	0.90
Whole-wheat pasta, cooked	1 cup	1.1*	0.23
Wild rice, cooked	1 cup	2.2	0.20
Fruits			
Apple, with skin	1	0.1	0.06
Avocado	1	0.8	0.53
Banana	1	0.2	0.12
Blueberries	1 cup	0.2	0.09
Cherries	1 cup	0.1	0.14
Dates	10	0.2	0.24
Fruit cocktail, in water	1/2 cup	0.1	0.09
Grapefruit	1/2	0.1	0.06
Grapes, green	1 cup	NA	0.26
Honeydew	1/10	NA	0.05
Nectarine	1	0.1	0.10
Orange	1	0.1	0.06

	Quantity	mg Zinc	mg Copper
Peach	1	0.1	0.06
Pear	1	0.2	0.19
Pineapple	1	0.1	0.17
Plum	1	0.1	0.03
Prune	10	0.5	0.36
Raisins, packed	1 cup	0.4	0.50
Raspberries	1 cup	0.6	0.09
Strawberries, fresh	1 cup	0.2	0.07
Tomato, canned	1/2 cup	0.2	0.14
Tomato, fresh	1	0.1	0.10
Watermelon	1 cup	0.1	0.05

Legumes

	Quantity	mg Zinc	mg Copper
Beans, refried	1 cup	3.5	1.04
Garbanzo beans, cooked	1 cup	2.5	0.58
Kidney beans, canned	1 cup	1.4	0.38
Kidney beans, cooked	1 cup	1.9	0.43
Lentils, cooked	1 cup	2.5	0.50
Lima beans, canned	1 cup	1.6	0.44
Navy beans, cooked	1 cup	1.9	0.54
Peas, split, cooked	1 cup	2.0	0.36
Pinto beans, cooked	1 cup	1.9	0.44
Soybeans, cooked	1 cup	1.9*	0.70

Meats

Beef

	Quantity	mg Zinc	mg Copper
Chuck roast	4 oz	11.6	0.17
Flank steak	4 oz	3.9	0.08
Ground beef, lean, broiled	3.5 oz	5.4	0.07
Heart	3 oz	2.7	0.63
Kidney	3.5 oz	4.2	0.68
Liver	4 oz	6.9	5.10
Rib roast	4 oz	4.1	0.07
Round steak	4 oz	3.4	0.08

	Quantity	mg Zinc	mg Copper
Sirloin steak	4 oz	3.9	0.09
Tenderloin	4 oz	5.6	0.18
Lamb			
Chops	4 oz	3.9	0.13
Leg of lamb	4 oz	5.7	0.14
Shoulder	4 oz	6.5	0.15
Luncheon Meat			
Chopped ham	1 slice	0.4	0.01
Frankfurter, beef/pork	1	0.8	0.04
Frankfurter, turkey	1	1.0	0.83
Turkey breast	1 slice	0.2	0.01
Turkey ham	2 slices	1.5	0.06
Pork			
Boneless ham, canned	3.5 oz	1.9	0.08
Leg, roasted	3.5 oz	2.9	0.10
Loin chop	1 chop	2.1	0.08
Veal			
Rib roast	4 oz	5.1	0.12
Wild Game			
Venison	4 oz	3.1	0.34

Nuts and Seeds

	Quantity	mg Zinc	mg Copper
Almond butter	1 Tbsp	0.5	0.14
Almonds, dry-roasted	1 oz	1.4	0.30
Brazil nuts	1 oz	1.3	0.50
Cashew butter	1 oz	1.5	0.62
Cashews, dry-roasted	1 oz	1.6	0.63
Coconut milk, raw	1 cup	1.6	0.64
Coconut, shredded	1 cup	0.9	0.37
Hazelnuts, dry-roasted	1 oz	0.7	0.44
Macadamia nuts	1 oz	0.5	0.08

	Quantity	mg Zinc	mg Copper
Mixed nuts, dry-roasted	1 oz	1.1	0.36
Peanut butter, chunky	2 Tbsp	0.9	0.17
Peanuts, dry-roasted	1 oz	0.9	0.19
Peanuts, Spanish, oil-roasted	1 oz	0.6	0.19
Pecans	1 oz	1.6	0.34
Pine nuts	1 oz	1.2	0.29
Pistachios	1 oz	0.4	0.34
Pumpkin seeds	1 oz	2.1	0.39
Soybeans, dry-roasted	1/2 cup	4.1*	0.93
Sunflower seeds	1 oz	1.4	0.50
Tahini sesame butter	1 Tbsp	0.7	0.24
Walnuts, black	1 oz	1.0	0.29
Walnuts, English	1 oz	0.8	0.39

Poultry

Chicken

	Quantity	mg Zinc	mg Copper
Dark w/o skin, roasted	3.5 oz	2.8	0.08
Giblets, simmered	3.5 oz	4.6	2.6
Light w/o skin, roasted	3.5 oz	1.2	0.05
Liver, simmered	3.5 oz	4.3	0.37
Whole w/o skin, stewed	3.5 oz	2.0	0.06

Duck

	Quantity	mg Zinc	mg Copper
Whole w/o skin, roasted	3.5 oz	2.6	0.23

Turkey

	Quantity	mg Zinc	mg Copper
Dark w/o skin, roasted	3.5 oz	4.5	0.16
Giblets, simmered	3.5 oz	3.7	0.39
Light w/o skin, roasted	3.5 oz	2.0	0.04

Snack Foods

	Quantity	mg Zinc	mg Copper
Corn chips	1 oz	0.4	0.04
Fruit leather	1 oz	0.0	0.04
Granola bar, plain	1 oz	0.6	0.11
Popcorn, air-popped	1 cup	0.3	0.03

	Quantity	mg Zinc	mg Copper
Pretzels	1 oz	0.2	0.09
Rice cakes, brown rice	1	0.3	0.04
Tortilla chips, plain	1 oz	0.4	0.03
Trail mix, regular	1 oz	0.9	0.28

Soups

Made with Milk

Clam chowder, New England	1 cup	0.8	0.14
Mushroom, cream of	1 cup	0.6	0.14
Oyster stew	1 cup	10.3	1.60
Pea, green	1 cup	1.8	0.39
Potato, cream of	1 cup	0.7	0.26
Tomato, cream of	1 cup	0.3	0.26

Made with Water

Black bean	1 cup	1.4	0.39
Chicken broth	1 cup	0.3	0.12
Chili, beef	1 cup	1.4	0.40
Miso	1 cup	9.2	1.21
Pea, split, w/ham	1 cup	1.3	0.37
Scotch broth	1 cup	1.6	0.25
Turkey-vegetable	1 cup	0.6	0.12

Vegetables

Artichoke hearts, boiled	1/2 cup	0.3	0.05
Asparagus, boiled	1/2 cup	0.4	0.09
Beets, cooked	1/2 cup	0.2	0.05
Black beans, cooked	1 cup	1.9	0.36
Broccoli, cooked	1/2 cup	0.1	0.05
Brussels sprouts, cooked	1/2 cup	0.3	0.07
Cabbage, boiled	1/2 cup	0.1	0.02
Carrots, cooked	1/2 cup	0.2	0.11
Carrots, raw	1 med	0.1	0.03
Cauliflower, cooked	1/2 cup	0.2	0.06

	Quantity	mg Zinc	mg Copper
Celery, raw	1/2 cup	0.1	0.02
Collards, cooked	1 cup	1.2	0.29
Corn, yellow, cooked	1/2 cup	0.4	0.04
Cucumber, raw	1 cup	0.2	0.04
Eggplant, cooked	1/2 cup	0.1	0.05
Green beans, cooked	1 cup	0.2	0.06
Kale, cooked	1/2 cup	0.2	0.10
Lettuce, iceberg	1 cup	0.3	0.04
Mixed vegetables, frozen	1/2 cup	0.5	0.08
Mushrooms, cooked	1/2 cup	0.7	0.39
Okra, cooked	1/2 cup	0.4	0.07
Onions, cooked	1/2 cup	0.2	0.04
Onions, green, raw	1/2 cup	0.2	0.03
Onions, mature, raw	1/2 cup	0.3	0.06
Parsnips, sliced, cooked	1/2 cup	0.2	0.11
Peas, green, cooked	1/2 cup	1.0	0.14
Peas and carrots, canned	1/2 cup	0.7	0.13
Pepper, chili, raw	1	0.1	0.08
Pepper, green, cooked	1/2 cup	0.1	0.05
Pepper, green, raw	1/2 cup	0.1	0.05
Pepper, jalapeño	1/2 cup	0.1	0.09
Pepper, red, raw	1/2 cup	0.1	0.05
Potato, baked w/skin	1 lg	0.6	0.62
Potato, boiled w/o skin	1	0.2	0.14
Potato, hash-browned	1/2 cup	0.3	0.14
Potato, mashed (homemade)	1/2 cup	0.8	0.20
Pumpkin, canned	1/2 cup	0.2	0.13
Seaweed, kelp	3.5 oz	1.2	0.28
Seaweed, wakame	3.5 oz	0.2	0.28
Spinach, cooked	1/2 cup	0.7	0.16
Squash, butternut	1/2 cup	0.1	0.07
Squash, spaghetti	1/2 cup	0.2	0.03
Succotash, cooked	1/2 cup	0.6	0.17
Sweet potato, baked	1	0.3	0.24
Water chestnuts, canned	1/2 cup	0.3	0.07
Yam, cooked	1/2 cup	0.1	0.10

	Quantity	mg Zinc	mg Copper
Yellow beans, cooked	1 cup	1.9	0.33
Zucchini, cooked	1/2 cup	0.2	0.08
Zucchini, raw	1/2 cup	0.1	0.04
Frozen Vegetables			
Chinese style	1/2 cup	0.2	0.04
Chow mein style	1/2 cup	0.2	0.10
Italian style	1/2 cup	0.2	0.06
Japanese style	1/2 cup	0.2	0.05
San Francisco style	1/2 cup	0.3	0.08
Stir-fry style	1/2 cup	0.3	0.09

Resources

Education

American Academy of Nutrition
3408 Sausalito Drive
Corona del Mar, CA 92625
800-290-4226
www.nutritioneducation.com

The American Academy of Nutrition is a great resource for individuals looking to learn more about nutrition in general and such subjects as nutritional counseling and female health concerns. The academy, which is accredited by the U.S. Department of Education Training Council, offers more than 20 home-study courses as well as a recently developed associate-of-science degree program in applied nutrition.

Rick Malter, Ph.D./Bloomingdale Counseling Services
148 S. Bloomingdale Road, Suite 112
Bloomingdale, IL 60108
630-894-4451

Dr. Rick Malter, director of Bloomingdale Counseling Services, has written several papers on copper toxicity that would be of particular interest to clinical psychologists. I was particularly impressed with two of his papers: "Copper Toxicity: Psychological Implications for Children, Adolescents, and Adults," and "Biochemistry and Psychodiagnostics: A Historical Perspective."

DESIGNS FOR HEALTH
211 PONDWAY LANE
TRUMBULL, CT 06611
203-371-4383
www.dfhi.com

Designs for Health is an educational institute and referral service that trains healthcare practitioners in cutting-edge clinical nutrition information, including how to properly interpret hair mineral analysis readings. Trainings, managed by nutritionists Linda Lizotte and Robert Crayhon, are held in the New York area as well as in Boulder, Colorado. A long-distance learning program is in the works. Interested healthcare practitioners should call for more information.

Food Products

MENTAL PROCESSES, INC.
1075 ZONOLITE RD., NE
ATLANTA, GA 30306
800-431-4018
www.pumpkorn.com
www.mentalprocesses.com

Mental Processes is the manufacturer of Pumpkorn, a delicious high-zinc snack food made out of pumpkin seeds. If you can't find this product in your local health-food store, you can call or visit the company's Web site and order the product directly.

Salivary Hormone Testing, Specialty Supplements, Products, Books, and Tissue Mineral Analysis

UNI KEY HEALTH SYSTEMS
P.O. BOX 7168
BOZEMAN, MT 59771
800-888-4353
www.unikeyhealth.com

Uni Key Health Systems is a great resource for meeting many needs. It now offers a special Evalu8 Test Kit that can be used to evaluate up to six hormones, including estradiol (the most potent of the estrogens), estriol (the safest of the estrogens), and progesterone. These hormones appear to be connected to copper-zinc balance in the body. Please call Uni Key customer service at 406-586-9424 for more information.

Uni Key has provided nutritional supplements and books to my clients and readers for more than six years. This company offers the female copper-free multiple-vitamin/mineral supplement that I developed specifically for women who have copper overload, as well as other formulas, such as one for adrenal gland support. The Doulton water filter, waterless cookware, and all of my books, including *Super Nutrition for Women, Super Nutrition for Menopause, Super Nutrition for Men,* and *Before the Change* also can be ordered through Uni Key. Call for a catalogue of all the latest products. If you'd like to get a tissue mineral analysis to determine your tissue copper levels, Uni Key can help provide this service for you. A typical analysis report is 6–12 pages in length and shows all major minerals as well as toxic metals including aluminum, lead, mercury, and copper. Recommendations are given for foods, diet, and supplements based upon individualized results.

Uni Key can also direct your health care practitioner to a tissue mineral lab. Have your practitioner call Uni Key.

Water Testing and Water Education

American Water Service
5001 Smith Farm Road
Matthews, NC 28105
800-788-4825
www.americanwaterservice.com

The American Water Service is a water education service and the manufacturer and distributor of affordable home water-testing kits that are easy to use, environmentally conscious, and based on EPA testing methods. The PurTest Iron Hardness Plus, which allows you to quickly and reliably test for copper and seven other factors in your water, retails for about $8. The PurTest Complete Home Water Analysis Kit, which allows you to check for 12 conditions and contaminants including copper, retails for about $30. You can call the company to order these products directly. After testing is complete, you can call the company for information and advice on how to best correct high levels of copper or other contaminants you may find in your water

Selected References

Adams, Ruth, and Frank Murray. *Minerals: Kill or Cure?* New York: Larchmont Books, 1974.

Aggett, Peter J., and Susan Fairweather-Tait. "Adaptation to High and Low Copper Intakes: Its Relevance to Estimated Safe and Adequate Daily Dietary Intakes." *American Journal of Clinical Nutrition* 67 (1998, suppl.): 1061S–1063S.

Balch, James F., and Phyllis A. Balch. *Prescription for Nutritional Healing,* 2nd ed. Garden City Park, NY: Avery, 1997.

Bennion, Lynn J., and others. "Effects of Oral Contraceptives on the Gallbladder Bile of Normal Women." *New England Journal of Medicine* 294, no. 4 (Jan. 22, 1976): 189–192.

Beshgetoor, Donna, and Michael Hambidge. "Clinical Conditions Altering Copper Metabolism in Humans." *American Journal of Clinical Nutrition* 67 (1998, suppl.): 1017S–1021S.

Bremner, Ian. "Manifestations of Copper Excess." *American Journal of Clinical Nutrition* 67 (1998, suppl.): 1069S–1073S.

"Cellular Uptake of Copper by Hepatocytes." *Nutrition Reviews* 49, no. 4 (Apr. 1991): 123–125.

Chatsworth, Colin, and Loren Chatsworth. *Energy: A Course on Increasing Your Energy Through the Balancing of Your Body's Minerals.* Charlottesville, VA: Healthview, 1985.

Chuong, C. James, and Earl B. Dawson. "Zinc and Copper Levels in Premenstrual Syndrome." *Fertility and Sterility* 62, no. 2 (Aug. 1994): 313–320.

"Copper-Glutathione: A Key Intermediate in Cellular Copper Metabolism?" *Nutrition Reviews* 49, no. 3 (Mar. 1991): 95–96.

Crayhon, Robert. *Robert Crayhon's Nutrition Made Simple*. New York: Evans, 1994.

Daweron, Charles T., and Mark D. Harrison. "Mechanisms for Protection Against Copper Toxicity." *American Journal of Clinical Nutrition* 67 (1998, suppl.): 1091S–1097S.

Eaton, S. B., S. B. Eaton III, and M. J. Konner. "Paleolithic Nutrition Revisited: A Twelve- Year Retrospective on Its Nature and Implications." *European Journal of Clinical Nutrition* 51 (1997): 207–216.

Eck, Paul C. "Insight into Copper Elimination." Phoenix, AZ: Eck Institute reference sheet, 1991.

———. "My Experiences with Copperheads." Phoenix, AZ: Eck Institute reference sheet, 1987.

Eck, Paul C., and Larry Wilson. "Adrenal Burnout Syndrome." Phoenix, AZ: Eck Institute reference sheet, 1989.

———. "Introduction to Copper Toxicity." Phoenix, AZ: Eck Institute reference sheet, 1987.

———. "Toxic Metals in Human Health and Disease." Phoenix, AZ: Eck Institute reference sheet (1989).

Fitzgerald, D. J. "Safety Guidelines for Copper in Water." *American Journal of Clinical Nutrition* 67 (1998, suppl.): 1098S–1120S.

Foreman, Debbie. "Vegetarianism: Is It the Right Choice?" Phoenix, AZ: Eck Institute reference sheet, 1987.

Gittleman, Ann Louise. *Before the Change: Taking Care of Your Perimenopause*. San Francisco: HarperSanFrancisco, 1998.

———. *Beyond Pritikin*. New York: Bantam Books, 1988.

———. *Super Nutrition for Menopause*. New York: Pocket Books, 1993.

———. *Super Nutrition for Women*. New York: Bantam Books, 1991.

———. *Your Body Knows Best*. New York: Pocket Books, 1996.

Ingelfinger, F. J. "Gallstones and Estrogens." *New England Journal of Medicine* 290, no. 1 (Jan. 3, 1974): 51–52.

Karcioglu, Zeynel A., and Rauf Sarper, eds. *Zinc and Copper in Medicine*. Springfield, IL: Charles C. Thomas, 1980.

Kirschmann, Gayla and John. *Nutrition Almanac Forth Edition*. New York: McGraw-Hill, 1996.

Levenson, Cathy W. "Mechanisms of Copper Conservation in Organs." *American Journal of Clinical Nutrition* 67 (1998, suppl.): 978S–981S.

Lizotte, Linda. "The Woman with Too Much Copper." *Total Health* 19, no. 4 (1997): 49.

Malter, Richard. "Copper Toxicity: Psychological Implications for Children, Adolescents, and Adults." Hoffman Estates, IL: A Malter Institute for Natural Development reference sheet, 1984.

———. "The Psychology of Energy, Stress, and Nutrition: New Concepts for Understanding Today's Health Trends." Hoffman Estates, IL: A Malter Institute for Natural Development reference sheet, 1993.

———. "Trace Mineral Analysis and Psychoneuroimmunology." *Townsend Letter for Doctors & Patients,* Apr. 1996, 50–62.

Martin, Jeanne Marie. "Overdosing on Copper?" *Alive* 62 (spring 1985): 43–44.

Nolan, Kevin R. "Copper Toxicity Syndrome." *Journal of Orthomolecular Psychiatry* 12, no. 4 (1983): 270–282.

Owen, Charles A., Jr. *Copper Deficiency and Toxicity: Acquired and Inherited, in Plants, Animals, and Man.* Park Ridge, NJ: Noyes Publications, 1981.

Packer, Lester, and others. "Alpha-Lipoic Acid as a Biological Antioxidant." *Free Radical Biology & Medicine* 19, no. 2 (1995): 227–250.

Passwater, Richard A. "Lipoic Acid Basics: An Interview with Dr. Clark." *Whole Foods,* Jan. 1996, pp. 49–53.

Passwater, Richard A., and Elmer M. Cranton. *Trace Elements, Hair Analysis, and Nutrition.* New Canaan, CT: Keats Publishing, 1983.

Pfeiffer, Carl C. *Mental and Elemental Nutrients.* New Canaan, CT: Keats Publishing, 1975.

———. *Nutrition and Mental Illness: An Orthomolecular Approach to Balancing Body Chemistry.* Rochester, VT: Healing Arts Press, 1987.

———. *Zinc and Other Micro-Nutrients.* New Canaan, CT: Keats Publishing, 1978.

Prasad, Ananda S. and Donald Oberlas, ed. *Biochemistry of Zinc.* New York: Plenum Press, 1993.

———, ed. *Trace Elements in Human Health and Disease.* Volume 1: *Zinc and Copper.* New York: Academic Press, 1976.

"Premenstrual Syndrome May Be Partly Linked to a Zinc Imbalance." *Better Nutrition,* July 1996, 12.

Schauss, Alexander, and Carolyn Costin. *Zinc and Eating Disorders.* New Canaan, CT: Keats Publishing, 1989.

Smith, Melissa Diane. "The Bad Side of Copper." *Let's Live,* Spring 1999 (to be published).

———. "Energy to Spare." *Delicious!* Apr. 1998, 32–36, 68–69.

———. "The Lowdown on Low Blood Sugar." *Delicious!* May 1998, 24, 26–27.

Turnlund, J. R., W. R. Keyes, G. L. Peiffer, and K. C. Scott. "Copper Absorption, Excretion, and Retention by Young Men Consuming Low Dietary Copper Determined by Using the Stable Isotope 65Cu." *American Journal of Clinical Nutrition* 67, no. 6 (1998): 1219–1225.

Vir, Sheila C., and others. "Serum and Hair Concentrations of Copper During Pregnancy." *American Journal of Clinical Nutrition* 34 (Nov. 1981): 2382–2388.

Watts, David L. "The Nutritional Relationships of Copper." *Journal of Orthomolecular Medicine* 4, no. 2 (1989): 99–108.

——. "The Nutritional Relationships of Zinc." *Journal of Orthomolecular Medicine* 3, no. 3 (1988): 63–67.

——. *Trace Elements and Other Essential Nutrients.* Dallas: Trace Elements, 1995.

Wilson, Lawrence. *Nutritional Balancing and Hair Mineral Analysis: A Comprehensive Guide.* Prescott, AZ: Wilson Consultants, 1991.

◆

For those of you who want to stay in touch with
Ann Louise Gittleman and learn more about her work,
schedule, and appearances in your area,
please see her Web Site: www.annlouise.com